Nurse Practitioner

Nurse Practitioner

Transition Guide

Sara L. Gleasman-DeSimone
Le Moyne College, Graduate
Nursing Department, Syracuse,
NY, USA

WILEY

Published by John Wiley & Sons, Inc., Hoboken, New Jersey.
Published simultaneously in Canada.

For general information on our other products and services or for technical support, please contact our Customer Care Department within the United States at (800) 762-2974, outside the United States at (317) 572-3993 or fax (317) 572-4002.

Wiley also publishes its books in a variety of electronic formats. Some content that appears in print may not be available in electronic formats. For more information about Wiley products, visit our web site at www.wiley.com.

Library of Congress Cataloging-in-Publication Data applied for

Paperback ISBN: 9781394303687

Cover Design: Wiley
Cover Image: © Sandipkumar Patel/Getty Images

Set in 11.5/14pt STIX Two Text by Straive, Pondicherry, India

Contents

Chapter 2   Certification and Career Preparation   19
Sara L. Gleasman-DeSimone PhD, ANP-C

Chapter 5 Launching Into Practice: The Inaugural Year 129
Sara L. Gleasman-DeSimone PhD, ANP-C

Contents

Chapter 8   Identifying Opportunities for Advancement   309

Sara L. Gleasman-DeSimone, PhD, ANP-C

Contents

List of Contributors

Therese Brown-Mahoney, MSN, CNM, NP
Le Moyne College, Graduate Nursing Department,
Syracuse, NY, USA

Deborah Clarey, FNP-C, RNFA
Mohawk Valley Health System, Oneida, NY, USA

Virginia Cronin, PhD, FNP-BC
Nascentia Health, Syracuse, NY, USA

Louise Dean-Kelly, PhD, DNS, FNP, RN
School of Nursing, State University of New York
Polytechnic Institute, Utica, New York, USA

Charles P. DeSimone, PhD
Upstate Medical University, Syracuse, NY, USA

Cynthia Grabski, DNS, FNP-BC
School of Nursing, State University of New York
Polytechnic Institute, Utica, NY, USA

Katherine Halstead, DNP, FNP-C
Le Moyne College, Graduate Nursing Department,
Syracuse, NY, USA

Mary Handley, PhD, LMHC, CRC
Le Moyne College, Clinical Mental Health Counseling
Program, Syracuse, NY, USA

Gina Myers, PhD, RN
Le Moyne College, Graduate Nursing Department,
Syracuse, NY, USA

Thomas J. Romano, MD
Gastroenterology & Hepatology of CNY, Liverpool,
NY, USA

Theresa Setter, APRN-BC, DCNP
Revitalize Dermatology & Aesthetics , Fayetteville,
NY, USA

Alyssa Sonneborn, FNP-BC
Le Moyne College, Syracuse, NY, USA

Martha Stevener, Practice Admistrator
Gastroenterology & Hepatology of CNY, Liverpool,
NY, USA

Colleen Zogby, FNP-C, PhD Candidate
Le Moyne College, Syracuse, NY, USA

Foreword

Dear Shiny New Nurse Practitioners (NPs),

I am honored to write the foreword to this very timely book, *Nurse Practitioner: Transition Guide*, by my friend and colleague Sara Gleasman-DeSimone. For several years, Sara and I collaborated in providing clinical services for an inpatient psychiatric unit and a comprehensive psychiatric emergency program. We also discussed cases and problems that needed to be addressed. I appreciated Sara's extensive knowledge base and sense of humor. As you can imagine, these patients presented many unique challenges in ascertaining and treating their medical problems.

I was employed as a registered nurse in various clinical settings before making a leap of faith and enrolling in an NP program. What followed was 35 years as an Adult NP, which included much independent administrative work. I have included some of this as a reminder that NPs must not only be clinically proficient, but they are likely to be in positions that require entirely new skills to promote the health and well-being of patients and the community. Chapter 7 of this book, Identifying Opportunities for Advancement of the NP, Specializations, Entrepreneurship, Quality Measures, and Outcomes, provides useful information in this regard.

- **My NP career began in the specialty of gynecology**: I was very grateful to the other NPs in the clinic for the teaching they provided to me. In addition to working in a free-standing clinic, I also served as the sole provider in two satellite clinics for other organizations.
- **Sole NP in a private radiation therapy practice**: In addition to medical care of patients, I also precepted NP students and supervised the medical portion of Radiation Therapy Technology students.
- **Four years at a National Institutes of Health-funded Chemosensory Disorders Clinic**: In addition to medical screening of patients, I contributed to policies, billing, and patient recruitment; case presentations to the research Project Director and Principal Investigators; and participated in olfactory and gustatory research projects.
- **Four years contracted to the Onondaga County Health Department Bureau of Disease Control**: Services included tuberculosis (TB) control, of which I was the director. I was responsible for clinical services, consultations for several other counties, grant writing, and budgets. I established a successful off-site clinic to test and screen newly arrived refugees for active and latent

TB infection. For two years, when I was the interim administrator of the Bureau, I also supervised the sexually transmitted disease (STD) clinic, employee health services, and reportable infectious diseases. I instituted cross-training of all employees, and made significant changes to the office space to facilitate this.

- **Occupational health services for a hospital and private companies**: Examinations, treatment of injuries, and employment clearances for a wide variety of occupations, such as truck drivers, law enforcement personnel, and HAZMAT workers; work site evaluations.

Chapters 2 and 5 are particularly helpful, since they describe methods of interviewing, patient-centered care, and professional practice guided by evidence. These become central to meeting new patients and establishing the beginnings of trust.

Everyone who contributed to the writing of this book remembers some trepidation when beginning the new role of an NP. In these pages you will see many suggestions for successful negotiation, networking, time management, and self-care, among others. I encourage you to fully engage with the content and apply the valuable lessons. It will make your transition from student to NP practice much easier.

The current landscape of NP practice is constantly evolving and improving. According to the American Association of Nurse Practitioners, Americans make nearly a billion visits to NPs each year, providing high-quality, patient-centered care. NPs can be found alleviating the primary care shortage in rural, urban, and suburban settings. I wish that I had this book when I started my career as an NP, and later as I changed positions. The principles never change. Patients want a well-educated NP who shows empathy, respect, and a willingness to work with other members of the care team. Congratulations to Sara for producing a book that should be required reading for all new NPs.

In closing, I would like to share with you the words my preceptorship coordinator, Mary Jean Thomas, told our class: "When you become an NP, your life will never be the same." I didn't know what she meant at the time, but looking back on everything I was able to bring to patients in this role, it made perfect sense.

Sincerely,

Elizabeth Belknap, RN, ANP

Elizabeth Belknap, ANP

Acknowledgments

I would like to express my gratitude to everyone who has supported me throughout the writing of this book. Your guidance, encouragement, and contributions have been invaluable and deeply appreciated.

I want to thank Charles, Sylvia, and Charlotte. Your support helped me meet the challenges and sacrifices required to write every day. Special thanks to Bean and Pesto for their "laptop support." To my parents, Genevieve and John, who instilled the value of education, and to my sisters Kelly and Lisa, for being a source of motivation and positivity.

To the contributing authors whom I deeply admire and intentionally invited to join this project: thank you for sharing your advice, stories, and expertise.

A special thanks to Tom, Christabel, Calee, Umar, Angelica, and all at Wiley for helping me navigate challenges with grace. Your resources and kind encouragement made a significant difference throughout this journey.

To my early mentors, Dr. Louise Dean-Kelly; Dr. Susan Bastable; Dr. Virginia Cronin; Debra Clarey, FNP; Katherine Mitchell RN, MSN, NP, and Barbara Carranti, CNS, who went above and beyond to support my teaching and practice. To Laureen Keegan, MSN, who played a pivotal role in helping me identify teachable moments and sharpen my critical thinking skills. To Dr. Mary Collins, Dr. Catherine Brownell, and Dr. Meega Wells for their leadership mentoring.

To Elizabeth Wright for helping me clear my path. Dr. Ferha Ternikar, thank you for modeling academic excellence and proving that writing a book is achievable. To Marisa Davis, OTD, for providing interprofessional education resources and always being kind and passionate about working with other disciplines.

Inspired by Dr. Loretta Ford, Dr. Elayne DeSimone, and Patricia Donnelly, FNP, who all helped blaze the trail for the nurse practitioner profession in various ways. Your influence runs deep.

To all nurse practitioners, seasoned and new, as well as my past and current students—this book is for you! It is my sincere hope that this work serves not only as a guide through the transition from student to nurse practitioner but also as a continued resource for your professional growth and success. Over the years as a nurse practitioner, I've witnessed the ongoing need for resources to address the challenges you face—whether it's contract negotiations, dealing with imposter syndrome, time management, or other issues related to transitioning into practice. We are lifelong learners, and this healthcare system relies on your expertise, innovation, and leadership to thrive. I wrote this book to guide you through it all and encourage continuous improvement.

I am proud to present this work to the nurse practitioner community. We are indeed a tight-knit group, bound together by a shared commitment to our patients. It is this bond that inspired every page of this book. Enjoy!

Chapter 1
Introduction

Sara L. Gleasman-DeSimone PhD, ANP-C

Le Moyne College, Graduate Nursing Department, Syracuse, NY, USA

1.1 Introduction

1.1.1 Transitions

Stepping out of the structured school environment and into independent clinical practice can feel overwhelming at first, especially without the guidance of a preceptor. For the new nurse practitioner (NP), understanding what to expect and how to navigate this shift can make a world of difference. During this time, one will begin forming a new professional identity and adopting a mindset aligned with the advanced nursing role.

1.1.2   Purpose

This book was created to support new NPs as they shift from their final semester of school to the challenges of their first year in practice. It aims to bridge the gap between classroom learning and the realities of professional work. It provides practical advice and strategies to make this period less over-whelming and more fulfilling. By blending actionable tips with academic insight, this guide equips new NPs with the tools and confidence they need to establish a strong foundation for a successful career.

1.2   Intended Audience

This book is developed for NP students in the final semester of their program and in the first year of practice. It also provides valuable insights for preceptors and faculty who play a crucial role in guiding new NPs, offering mentorship, support, and practical advice to help them integrate success-fully into their roles.

1.3   Importance of Book

1.3.1   Growth of the Profession

The NP profession continues to experience significant growth. As of November 2023, there are approximately 385,000 licensed NPs in the United States, marking an

8.5% increase from 355,000 in 2022 [1]. This steady growth reflects the rising demand for high-quality, patient-centered care, which NPs deliver across diverse settings. A key driver of this expansion is the NPs' ability to address healthcare shortages and improve access to care, particularly in underserved areas. Legislative advancements in many states have granted full practice authority (FPA) to NPs, enabling them to practice independently. These changes highlight the recognition of NPs as providers of high-quality, cost-effective care. Furthermore, the expansion of Doctor of Nursing Practice (DNP) programs equips NPs to apply evidence-based practices in clinical settings to improve patient outcomes.

On a global scale, the role of NPs is also expanding. For example, the American Association of Nurse Practitioners (AANP) launched an international membership category in 2024, reflecting the global growth of advanced practice nursing. The AANP supports the international NP community through initiatives like the International Advanced Practice Nurse Ambassador Program, which funds international participants' attendance at AANP conferences to foster collaboration and learning. Additionally, the organization collaborates with global partners to advance NP roles and improve patient access to care worldwide [2]. These efforts demonstrate the profession's adaptability and growing influence on healthcare systems across various regions.

Looking ahead, the US Bureau of Labor Statistics projects a 45% increase in NP employment from 2022 to 2032, a growth rate significantly higher than the average for all occupations [3]. This rapid expansion is driven by escalating healthcare demands, an aging population, and provider shortages.

However, NPs have earned top recognition in US News & World Report's 2024 rankings, securing the titles of Best Job,

Best Healthcare Job, and Best STEM Job [4]. This acclaim highlights the profession's ability to deliver cost-effective, high-quality primary care. Efforts by organizations like the AANP to expand and diversify the workforce will help sustain this growth and ensure that NPs continue to meet the needs in the healthcare environment [1].

1.4 Historical Background of Nurse Practitioner Practice

1.4.1 The Beginning

The NP profession began with a vision to train nurses to provide advanced care. This idea came to fruition in 1965 when Dr. Loretta Ford and Dr. Henry Silver established the first NP program at the University of Colorado. Their goal was to expand the role of nurses by integrating advanced clinical skills with a focus on disease prevention and health promotion. This innovative program enabled nurses to assume advanced roles in providing primary care, particularly to underserved populations, laying the foundation for the NP profession [5]. Shortly thereafter, Boston College introduced a graduate-level NP program, and by 1973, more than 65 NP programs were operational across the United States. That same year, the National Association of Pediatric Nurse Practitioners (NAPNAP) was founded, playing a critical role in advancing pediatric healthcare.

1.4.2 Definition and Growth of the Profession

As the years went on, there was continued growth for NP programs as the profession gained broader recognition. By 1989, 90% of NP programs were offering master's degrees or higher, reflecting the profession's commitment to advanced education and professionalization [6]. The AANP, established in 1983 with just 100 members, became a cornerstone of professional advocacy. By launching its journal in 1989, the AANP provided NPs with a dedicated platform to share research and best practices that further formalized the profession. By the end of the 2000s, the number of practicing NPs in the United States had surpassed 130,000, underscoring the growing role of NPs as essential healthcare providers.

1.4.3   Evolving Policy and Practice

Around this time, many states passed laws to formally define the NP role and give them greater independence in practice [7]. These legal milestones created a foundation for the profession's growth, opening the door to expanded responsibilities and authority. For example, the Balanced Budget Act of 1997 increased reimbursement for NP services under Medicare and Medicaid, solidifying the NP role as providers in the healthcare system [6]. This ensured reimbursement equity at 85% of the physician rate for equivalent services. Additionally, the Affordable Care Act (ACA) emphasized team-based, patient-centered care models, such as patient-centered medical homes and accountable care organizations, where NPs play a pivotal role in delivering primary care.

One of the most significant advancements for NPs is FPA. With FPA, NPs can independently practice without the need for physician oversight. This change is important for addressing healthcare challenges like improving access to care in underserved areas. This also meets the growing demand created by an aging population and the rise in chronic diseases [6]. By 2023, 27 states and the District of Columbia had adopted FPA, with more states working toward similar legislation. However, NPs deliver care that matches and sometimes exceeds that of physicians in areas like patient outcomes, satisfaction, and cost-effectiveness [8]. The COVID-19 pandemic underscored the autonomy and flexibility of NPs, as many states temporarily relaxed physician supervision requirements, strengthening the case for making FPA a permanent policy. Policy advancements have not only expanded NP autonomy but also highlighted the importance of supporting novice NPs during their transition to independent practice [8, 9].

1.5 What Do You Call a Nurse Practitioner?

The terminology used to describe NPs can significantly impact their professional identity and perception within healthcare. Terms like "midlevel provider" and "physician extender" are often viewed as demeaning and have been associated with discomfort and professional conflict [10]. Despite their use in some settings to differentiate NPs from physicians, these labels fail to reflect the expertise and autonomy of NPs. It is recommended to use appropriate professional titles that recognize their qualifications, particularly for those holding a doctoral degree [11]. Using respectful and accurate terminology not only validates the NP role but also fosters greater collaboration within healthcare teams.

1.6 Elevator Speech

An elevator speech is a concise summary that communicates an NP's role and value. This helps NPs confidently highlight their expertise, build connections, and advocate for their profession in various settings. However, NPs are advanced practice registered nurses with graduate or doctoral-level education who assess, diagnose, treat, and prescribe medications. They provide primary, acute, and specialty healthcare, focusing on health promotion and disease prevention. This focus on disease prevention helps improve overall health outcomes and reduces the burden of preventable illnesses [12]. Furthermore, NPs work closely with interdisciplinary teams, contributing their expertise to improve communication and coordination, ultimately enhancing patient outcomes [13].

The AANP defines NPs as "licensed, autonomous clinicians who blend clinical expertise in diagnosing and treating health conditions with a focus on disease prevention and health promotion" [14]. This evidence-based, patient-centered approach underscores their essential role in healthcare.

1.7 Challenges Influencing Practice

The expanding role of NPs has brought heightened expectations and responsibilities, particularly for new graduates transitioning into practice. This period often presents significant challenges that can negatively impact confidence, job satisfaction, and retention [15]. For novice NPs, bridging the gap between academic preparation and professional reality frequently becomes a source of stress. This transitional phase can hinder role development, increase turnover intentions, and ultimately jeopardize the stability of the healthcare workforce [15].

One common challenge for new NPs is unclear role definitions and inadequate onboarding processes, which contribute to feelings of uncertainty and frustration. These stressors are further exacerbated by the emotional burden of managing changing conditions and meeting the expectations of others. Such pressures create additional hurdles during the adjustment period. This can complicate the transition [16].

Novice NPs face internal challenges, including low confidence and limited meaningful patient interactions, which can reduce job satisfaction. Without support, these issues may hinder growth, lower self-efficacy, and increase isolation [15]. Moreover, balancing personal and professional responsibilities while striving to maintain work-life balance adds another layer of complexity to this phase.

1.8   Support of Practice

To address the challenges faced by novice NPs, healthcare organizations should implement tailored support systems. This can foster confidence and professional development. Structured onboarding processes, role-specific training programs, and clear role definitions can significantly reduce uncertainty and anxiety. By setting clear expectations and providing consistent guidance, organizations can enhance novice NPs' confidence and job satisfaction [15].

Mentorship programs serve as a strategy for supporting new NPs. Experienced mentors provide guidance, share valuable insights, and offer support that helps novice practitioners navigate their professional growth. These relationships can reduce feelings of isolation, bolster self-efficacy, and improve both job satisfaction and long-term retention [15].

In addition to organizational initiatives, intrinsic motivators play a vital role in fostering professional fulfillment. A sense of purpose, meaningful patient interactions, and opportunities for skill development enhance job satisfaction. In addition, examining extrinsic factors, such as competitive compensation and flexible schedules, is equally important in promoting work-life balance. This can help reduce burnout. By alleviating external stressors, these measures allow NPs to focus on their roles without feeling overwhelmed [15]. Adapting to the demands of an expanded role requires both individual effort and organizational commitment. When novice NPs are equipped with adequate resources, mentorship, and structural support, they are more likely to succeed and contribute to a stable and effective healthcare workforce [16].

1.9 Setting Realistic Goals and Expectations

Graduating from an accredited program with many clinical hours and didactic learning provides a strong foundation, but the first year of practice often presents a steep learning curve. This phase requires patience, resilience, and realistic goal setting. Encountering challenges and unfamiliar situations is inevitable [17]. While uncertainty and self-doubt are natural during this transition, acknowledging these feelings can be validating [18]. Building connections with colleagues and former instructors can offer support, encouragement, and perspective. This can help new NPs adjust their expectations during this period.

One way the NP can grow professionally is through reflection. Reflection is a powerful tool that enables NPs to thoughtfully evaluate their experiences, celebrate successes, and identify areas for improvement. Techniques such as journaling, seeking feedback, and engaging in peer discussions foster deeper engagement with the role and promote continuous development [19]. Structured plans and clear timelines provide direction and momentum for achieving both short- and long-term objectives. By embracing reflection and setting realistic goals, NPs can confidently navigate the challenges of their first year and build a strong foundation for success.

1.10   Introduction to the Nurse Practitioner Transitions to Practice Guidebook

The role of the NP has evolved considerably over recent years. As healthcare systems grow more complex and patient needs become more diverse, NPs are positioned at the forefront of transformative care. This guidebook is designed to serve as a comprehensive roadmap for new and emerging NPs, offering insight into the critical skills, competencies, and knowledge areas essential for success in transition to practice.

1.11   Structure and Overview

This book is structured to provide both a linear journey through professional development and a reference tool for specific challenges NPs may encounter. Each chapter builds on the previous one, beginning with fundamental job essentials and culminating in self-care strategies and pathways for career advancement. This progression mirrors the typical experience of a new NP, addressing both the concerns of finding a job and the long-term considerations for career sustainability and growth.

1.11.1 Chapters 1–3: Building a Foundation for Nurse Practitioner Career Success

The three opening chapters of this guidebook lay the groundwork for new NPs to transition confidently into the workforce. They cover three essential pillars: career preparation, job acquisition, and professional negotiation. The first chapter, Certification and Job Essentials for the NP, focuses on obtaining certification and developing a clear and authentic professional identity. Readers are guided through creating tailored resumes and cover letters that highlight their unique qualifications and skills. This chapter also offers networking strategies and the strategic use of online platforms to expand professional connections. Next, Interview Mastery for the NP equips readers with the tools to approach job interviews with confidence and precision. This chapter offers practical advice on presenting oneself as both clinically competent and personable, showcasing expertise and interpersonal strengths. It explores common interview questions, scenario-based discussions, and key preparation strategies. The third chapter, Contract Negotiation Skills, tackles the often overlooked yet vital skill of understanding and negotiating employment terms. Contract negotiation can be daunting for new NPs, but this chapter simplifies the process, providing clear guidance on interpreting key terms and strategies for negotiating salaries, benefits, and raises. By mastering these skills, NPs can confidently advocate for equitable compensation and benefits.

Together, these chapters provide a comprehensive roadmap for new NPs, emphasizing the importance of self-presentation, preparation, and assertiveness. By addressing these foundational elements, this guide empowers readers to navigate the transition into practice with confidence and build a successful, long-term professional journey.

1.11.2 Chapter 4: Launching into Practice: The Inaugural Year

Chapter 4 focuses on effective onboarding, credentialing, and understanding legal and regulatory constraints. This is to ensure a smooth integration into clinical practice. The chapter introduces strategies to build clinical competence through experiential learning and Patricia Benner's "Novice to Expert" framework, advocating for reflective practices and mentorship. It addresses challenges like imposter syndrome, offering practical solutions to bolster confidence and resilience. Additionally, the chapter underscores the necessity of time management and organizational support to enhance efficiency, professional growth, and job satisfaction, ultimately ensuring high-quality patient care.

1.11.3 Chapter 5: Patient-Centered Care

Chapter 5 delves into patient-centered care, the cornerstone of NP practice. It focuses on how empathy, therapeutic communication, and cultural competence can build trust and enhance patient outcomes. The chapter explores the role of self-efficacy, motivational interviewing, and evidence-based practice. This content assists in making thoughtful clinical decisions and encouraging meaningful behavioral changes in patients. In addition, it emphasizes the importance of ethical principles and fostering diversity, equity, and inclusion (DEI) to create an inclusive healthcare environment.

Readers will find practical strategies for handling difficult patient interactions, applying motivational theories, and navigating ethical challenges. By blending clinical expertise with a deep respect for individual patient preferences, this chapter aims to empower NPs to provide truly patient-centered care.

1.11.4 Chapter 6: Self-Care

Chapter 6 highlights the importance of self-care for NPs as a foundation for maintaining competence, resilience, and job satisfaction. It presents self-care not just as a personal choice but as an ethical responsibility within the nursing profession, emphasizing its role in reducing burnout, compassion fatigue, and workplace stress. The chapter introduces practical tools, such as self-care assessments, to help NPs develop personalized strategies for overall well-being. It also explores the importance of resilience and emotional intelligence, which are critical for navigating the challenges of practice. Readers will discover actionable interventions, including mindfulness practices, boundary-setting techniques, and the benefits of peer support. The chapter calls on healthcare systems to prioritize self-care alongside individual efforts, supporting its necessity for sustaining professional well-being and enhancing patient outcomes.

1.11.5 Chapter 7: Identifying Opportunities for Advancement

This final chapter focuses on key areas that shape the evolving role of NPs' specialization, recertification, mentorship, and emerging trends. It highlights the wealth of opportunities for NPs to advance their careers through continuing education, obtaining specialized certifications, and stepping into leadership roles. The chapter emphasizes the importance of staying adaptable in a rapidly changing healthcare environment such as artificial intelligence (AI). It explores various pathways for career growth, including pursuing specializations, engaging in quality improvement initiatives, and obtaining terminal degrees like the DNP.

In addition, this chapter discusses initiatives aimed at expanding the NP role, reducing healthcare disparities, and fostering stronger interprofessional collaboration. Through real-world examples and practical strategies, it encourages NPs to embrace innovation, hone their leadership skills, and make meaningful contributions to healthcare systems. By blending insights on career development with actionable advice, this chapter serves as both a guide and an inspiration for NPs to take their practice to the next level.

1.12   Learning Activities

This book incorporates a variety of learning activities designed to engage students, stimulate critical thinking, and promote professional growth. Each chapter begins with clear objectives to guide the learner's focus and goals. Case studies simulate real-world clinical scenarios, ethical dilemmas, and interprofessional collaboration, offering a realistic perspective on NP practice while encouraging critical thinking and problem-solving. Reflection exercises prompt students to examine their professional growth, ethical responsibilities, and the cultural dimensions of patient care, fostering deeper self-awareness and empathy. Personalized planning activities support students in developing tailored goals for continuing education and certifications, aligning their learning with long-term career aspirations.

These activities are adaptable across different educational formats, making them ideal for NP programs in both traditional classroom settings and virtual learning environments. In-person programs can use case studies and group discussions to spark peer collaboration, while online platforms enable interactive simulations, discussion boards, and reflective journaling. Competency-based assessments and rubric-based grading ensure consistent evaluation standards. By incorporating these comprehensive strategies, this book creates a learner-centered experience.

1.13   Conclusion

This book takes a holistic approach to addressing the evolving challenges of post-COVID healthcare and the unique experiences of NPs. Through personal stories, interactive case studies, and reflection exercises, it connects readers with the real-world journeys of recent graduates and seasoned professionals. These elements provide practical insights while offering reassurance that the transition from novice to expert is a shared experience.

In addition to practical guidance, the book fosters a sense of community. It includes networking strategies and tips for utilizing social media to remain connected with the broader NP field, supporting and inspiring practitioners as they grow in their roles.

At its core, this book aims to empower NPs by equipping them with the confidence, resilience, and purpose needed to succeed. With the tools and strategies outlined, practitioners

will be prepared to embrace opportunities, overcome challenges, and continue growing as dynamic leaders in the
evolving landscape of healthcare!

References

1. American Association of Nurse Practitioners (2023). Nurse practitioner profession grows to 385,000 strong. https://www.aanp.
   org/news-feed/nurse-practitioner-profession-grows-
   to-385-000-strong (accessed 12 December 2023).
2. Ferrara, S.A. (2024). Nurse practitioners around the world.
   J. Nurse Pract. 1: https://doi.org/10.1016/j.nurpra.
   2024.105246.
3. U.S. Bureau of Labor Statistics (2023). A look at nurse practitioners for National Nurse Practitioner Week. https://www.bls.
   gov/opub/ted/2023/a-look-at-nurse-practitioners-
   for-national-nurse-practitioner-week.htm (accessed
   20 November 2023).
4. Ferrara, S.A. (2024). The future is bright for nurse practitioners.
   J. Nurse Pract. 20(1): 1. https://doi.org/10.1016/j.nurpra.
   2024.104948.
5. Ford, L. and Silver, H. (1967). *The Origins of Nurse Practitioner
   Practice: A New Direction in Nursing and Medicine.* University
   of Colorado.
6. American Association of Nurse Practitioners (AANP) (2023).
   State practice environment. www.aanp.org (accessed
   9 November 2023).
7. Pulcini, J., Jelic, M., Gul, R., and Loke, A.Y. (2010). An international survey on advanced practice nursing education, practice,
   and regulation. *J. Nurs. Scholarsh.* 42 (1): 31–39. https://doi.
   org/10.1111/j.1547-5069.2009.01322.x.
8. National Academy of Medicine (2021). *The Future of Nursing
   2020–2030: Charting a Path to Achieve Health Equity.* National
   Academies Press.
9. Centers for Medicare & Medicaid Services (2022). Medicare
   reimbursement for nurse practitioners. www.cms.gov (accessed
   12 December 2023).

10. American Association of Nurse Practitioners (AANP) (2022). Use of terms such as mid-level provider and physician extender. https://www.aanp.org/advocacy/advocacy-resource/position-statements/useof-terms-such-as-mid-level-provider-and-physician-extender (accessed 12 December 2023).
11. Beasley, L.D. (2024). The titles we use matter. *J. Nurse Pract.* 105027. https://doi.org/10.1016/j.nurpra.2024.105027.
12. Bodenheimer, T. and Bauer, L. (2016). Rethinking the primary care workforce—an expanded role for nurse practitioners. *N. Engl. J. Med.* 375 (23): 2245–2247.
13. Bauer, L. (2010). Nurse practitioners as an underutilized resource for health reform: evidence-based demonstrations of cost-effectiveness. *J. Am. Assoc. Nurse Pract.* 22 (4): 228–231.
14. American Association of Nurse Practitioners (AANP). What's a nurse practitioner (NP)? AANP Website (accessed 2022).
15. Barnes, H., Faraz Covelli, I., and Rubright, R. (2022). The transition from novice to practicing nurse practitioner: challenges and factors influencing retention. *J. Nurs. Scholarsh.* 54 (1): 38–45.
16. Cheng, J.F., Wang, T.J., Huang, X.Y., and Han, H.C. (2022). First-year experience of transitioning from registered nurse to nurse practitioner. *J. Am. Assoc. Nurse Pract.* 34 (8): 978–990. https://doi.org/10.1097/JXX.0000000000000750. PMID: 36330551.
17. Morris, G. (2023). What no one tells you as a new NP grad. NurseJournal. https://nursejournal.org (accessed 24 November 2024).
18. Barnes, H. (2015). Exploring the factors that influence nurse practitioner role transition. *J. Nurse Pract.* 11 (2): 178–183. https://doi.org/10.1016/j.nurpra.2014.11.004. PMID: 25685113; PMCID: PMC4323084.
19. Koshy, K., Limb, C., Gundogan, B. et al. (2017). Reflective practice in health care and how to reflect effectively. *Int. J. Surg. Oncol.* 2 (6): e20. https://doi.org/10.1097/IJ9.0000000000000020. Epub 2017 Jun 15. PMID: 29177215; PMCID: PMC5673148.

Chapter 2
Certification and Career Preparation

Sara L. Gleasman-DeSimone PhD, ANP-C

Le Moyne College, Graduate Nursing Department, Syracuse, NY, USA

From Passion to Practice
Thomas J. Romano, MD

Nurse Practitioner: Transition Guide, First Edition. Sara L. Gleasman-DeSimone.
© 2025 John Wiley & Sons, Inc. Published 2025 by John Wiley & Sons, Inc.

Chapter Highlights

Certification
Licensing
Job Search
Resume
Cover Letter
Professional Identity
Networking

2.1   Introduction

Starting a career as a nurse practitioner (NP) involves more than mastering clinical and didactic skills. It also means navigating certification requirements, planning a focused job search, and building a strong professional presence. For many, the process begins as early as admission to an NP program, when initial ideas about career paths start to form. These ideas often shift and develop further through clinical rotations and hands-on experiences. Certification plays a pivotal role in the transition from a student to a practicing NP. It validates one's clinical expertise and ensures alignment with the chosen specialty area. This chapter provides a comprehensive guide to certification and licensing, along with practical advice for crafting effective resumes and cover letters. It also offers tips on creating a positive professional image, helping new NPs present themselves confidently.

With 45 years in the medical field, I have had the privilege of seeing countless nurses choose to advance their careers and pursue the role of an NP. It is not only intelligence that

Objectives with Mapping to 2021 AACN Masters Essentials

Apply knowledge of NP certification requirements. Mapped to Domain 9: Professionalism

Identify key components of an NP resume and cover letter. Mapped to Domain 9: Professionalism

Analyze various job search strategies and networking methods. Mapped to Domain 9 10: Personal, Professional, and Leadership Development

Develop a professional online profile and social media presence. Mapped to Domain 8: Informatics and Healthcare Technologies

Create a tailored resume and cover letter that effectively highlight skills, achievements, and certifications relevant to specific NP job applications. Mapped to Domain 9: Professionalism

has brought you here but also a genuine love for what you do. After finishing your clinicals, you likely have a strong sense of what you enjoy and where your strengths lie. Let this knowledge and confidence guide you as you navigate the first steps of your career. Focus on making your resume clear and concise. Employers seek candidates who are hardworking, efficient, and, most importantly, love what they do. When you bring that passion to your role, it resonates with patients and colleagues alike, creating a positive environment throughout the organization. Yes, it is that easy! Enjoy the journey!

2.1.1   State Licensing and National Certification

State licensing and national certification are two distinct steps required for NPs to begin their professional practice. State licensure is specific to the state where the NP intends to work and serves as legal authorization to practice [1]. It involves meeting state-specific requirements. In contrast, national certification is a standardized process that verifies an NP's clinical knowledge and expertise in a specialty area, such as family nurse practitioner (FNP). Certification is achieved by passing a national certification exam. These exams are administered by recognized organizations like the American Nurses Credentialing Center (ANCC) and the American Academy of Nurse Practitioners Certification Board (AANPCB) [2, 3]. While certification validates clinical competence at a national level, state licensure establishes the legal framework for practice within a specific jurisdiction.

2.1.1.1   State Forms

Each state can differ in requirements for licensure. For example, to become a licensed NP in New York State, an applicant must hold a New York State RN license. If they are not yet licensed in that state as a registered nurse, they should first apply through the New York State Education Department (NYSED) [1]. Next, the NP Certification Application, or Form 1—Application for Licensure, must be submitted online with an $85 fee covering both the application and initial registration. This application includes sections for personal information, education, and professional experience.

Following this, the applicant's educational institution must send Form 2, which confirms education completed to the NYSED. The student completes section one of this form. This form is then sent to the school and filled out by the registrar's office. After the school completes their part on Form 2, it is sent to the NYSED email or to their physical address. This certifies successful completion of the program. If the applicant's program did not include pharmacotherapeutics coursework covering state and federal laws, they would complete this training through an approved provider. That provider would submit Form 2B. If the program included this coursework, then this form is not necessary. If the applicant is certified by a national certifying organization, then they should request the organization to send Form 3, Verification of National Nurse Practitioner Examination, directly to the NYSED [1].

Additionally, in New York State, newly graduated NPs have fewer than 3,600 hours of experience. They are required to establish a collaborative practice agreement with a physician. The applicant should complete Form 4NP, Verification of Collaborative Agreement and Practice Protocol, and submit it to the NYSED within 90 days of beginning practice. This does not need to be done at the time of licensing. Upon completion of all forms and fees, NYSED reviews the application, and if approved, issues NP certification, allowing the individual to practice within New York State. This can take up to 6–12 weeks. To access the required forms, visit the NYSED Office of the Professions website at www.op.nysed.gov [1]. While this example outlines the process for New York State, applicants should review the specific requirements and procedures for the state in which they plan to practice in.

2.1.1.2 National Certification

In the United States, NPs can pursue various types of certifications, each aligned with their specialty area. To ensure NPs meet the highest standards of competence and professionalism, several certification bodies offer specialized certification programs. The ANCC, the AANPCB, the Pediatric Nursing Certification Board (PNCB), and other specialty certification boards detail their requirements and processes [2, 3].

A chart of common certifications and what organization offers certification is shown as follows.

Certifications and Certification Bodies

NP Certification	Certification Body	Additional Notes
Family Nurse Practitioner (FNP)	American Nurses Credentialing Center (ANCC), American Academy of Nurse Practitioners Certification Board (AANPCB)	Care across the lifespan
Adult-Gerontology Primary Care NP (AGPCNP)	ANCC, AANPCB	Focuses on adolescents to elderly
Adult-Gerontology Acute Care NP (AGACNP)	ANCC	Focuses on acute care for adults

NP Certification	Certification Body	Additional Notes
Pediatric Nurse Practitioner (PNP)	The Pediatric Nursing Certification Board (PNCB) ANCC	Specializes in pediatric care
Psychiatric Mental Health Nurse Practitioner (PMHNP)	ANCC	Specializes in mental healthcare across the lifespan
Women's Health Nurse Practitioner (WHNP)	The National Certification Corporation (NCC)	Focuses on reproductive and gynecologic health
Neonatal Nurse Practitioner (NNP)	NCC	Specializes in neonatal intensive care
Emergency Nurse Practitioner (ENP)	AANPCB	For FNPs providing emergency care

American Academy of Nurse Practitioners (AANP)

The AANPCB offers several national certifications for NPs, each focusing on various specialties [2]. The FNP certification tests clinical knowledge for care across the lifespan, from prenatal to older adults. The Adult-Gerontology Primary Care Nurse Practitioners (AGNP) certification focuses on adolescents through elder adults, and those who are dually certified as both Adult Nurse Practitioners (ANP) and Gerontology Nurse Practitioners (GNP) can apply to convert their certification to AGNP. For those in emergency care, the Emergency Nurse Practitioner (ENP) certification is available for FNPs meeting specific eligibility criteria. This certification was developed in collaboration with the American Academy of Emergency Nurse Practitioners (AAENP) in 2016. It was designed to further define the role of FNPs who provide emergency care across all age groups and levels of acuity. At last, the Psychiatric Mental Health Nurse Practitioner (PMHNP) certification tests entry-level clinical competency in psychiatric care across the lifespan. Each certification ensures that NPs meet high standards of care in their respective specialties [4].

American Nurses Credentialing Center

The ANCC provides several specialization options, including PMHNP-BC, Adult-Gerontology Primary Care Nurse Practitioner (AGPCNP-BC), Adult-Gerontology Acute Care Nurse Practitioner (AGACNP-BC), and FNP-BC [3].

AANP and American Nurses Credentialing Center Testing

Both the AANPCB and the ANCC have an application process to test in their specialty [2, 3]. Candidates must have a graduate degree from an accredited NP program for that specialty. After graduating and completing the required clinical practice hours, they are eligible to test to obtain national certification in their specialty area. Once their education, clinical hours, and RN licensure are confirmed, they can schedule the exam. Both certification bodies administer their exams as computer-based tests, using multiple-choice questions to assess advanced clinical skills and knowledge.

The Pediatric Nursing Certification Board

The PNCB is a leading organization certifying Pediatric Nurse Practitioners (PNPs) to ensure they meet high standards in pediatric care [5]. Candidates for PNCB certification must have a graduate degree from an accredited pediatric NP program, hold national certification, and complete a required number of clinical practice hours. The PNCB certification exam is computer-based and focuses specifically on pediatric care. Steps to certification include completing an accredited program, gaining pediatric clinical experience, obtaining national certification, and passing the PNCB exam [5].

Within pediatric care, Acute Care Certified Pediatric Nurse Practitioners (CPNP-AC) are specialists trained to manage complex and critical health issues in young patients. They work collaboratively with interdisciplinary teams to provide care for patients experiencing severe and acute health conditions. On the other hand, Primary Care Certified Pediatric Nurse Practitioners (CPNP-PC) play a crucial role in preventive care, managing common acute and chronic conditions, and promoting overall well-being through family and community-based care approaches. Additionally, Pediatric Primary Care Mental Health Specialists (PMHS) address the rising demand for mental health services among youth, managing conditions such as depression, anxiety, and autism to improve access to emotional and cognitive healthcare [5].

2.1.1.3   Certification Review Courses

While taking a review course for NP certification is often optional, it can be highly beneficial by providing structured study materials and guidance. These courses cover essential content from the entire program and often include a comprehensive exam to identify strengths and weaknesses. This allows students and graduates to focus their study efforts where they are needed most. Typical course features include practice questions, detailed content reviews, and test-taking strategies, all designed to reinforce understanding and improve retention of complex material. By pinpointing areas for improvement, review courses help candidates get the most out of study time, build confidence, and increase their chances of passing the certification exam on the first attempt. Given these benefits, selecting the right review course for that individual becomes an important step in preparing for success.

When choosing a review course, it is important to consider personal learning preferences and practical needs. For example, a self-paced course may suit those who prefer studying on their own schedule, while a live course could benefit individuals who need real-time interaction and support. Time availability is another factor as some may require an intensive, short-term course to fit within limited study windows. Others might prefer a gradual, in-depth learning process. Online courses offer flexibility for those unable to attend in person, while budget constraints should also guide the decision. Consider potential additional fees for materials like study guides or practice exams and look for value-added options such as free retakes or early registration discounts.

For those needing extra support in specific areas, such as pharmacology or pathophysiology, tailored courses and supplemental materials such as flashcards and online tests can help with preparation. Access to instructor support or an online community adds another layer of assistance, ensuring candidates stay on track. Finally, researching a course's reputation, including pass rates and testimonials from past students, can help. By carefully evaluating these factors, NP candidates can select a review course that aligns with their needs and optimizes their preparation for certification success.

Examples of Review Courses

Provider	Description	Website
APEA (Advanced Practice Education Associates)	Offers a range of review courses in multiple formats, including live, webinar, and on-demand options, with comprehensive resources for NP certification preparation	`https://apea.com/courses/`
Fitzgerald Health Education	Provides in-depth NP review courses with various formats to support exam preparation, including extensive study materials and practice resources	`https://www.fhea.com/np-certification-exam-review`

(continued)

Provider	Description	Website
American Nurses Association (ANA)	Delivers online NP review courses, focusing on certification preparation and continuing education credits	`https://www.nursingworld.org/continuing-education/ce-subcategories/certification-review/`
Kaplan Test Prep	Offers self-paced, on-demand NP review courses with access to practice questions, videos, and structured study plans	`https://www.kaptest.com/nurse-practitioner`
Sarah Michelle NP Reviews	Provides self-paced online courses and live study groups, along with access to a supportive online community for exam preparation	`https://www.npreviews.com/`

However, NPs are required to fulfill continuing education requirements to maintain their certification, ensuring they stay current with advancements in clinical practice and patient care. Recertification is further discussed in Chapter 7.

2.1.2 Job Preparation

Newly credentialed NPs can embark on their job search, ready to apply their specialized skills across diverse employment opportunities. While some may have begun preparing during their training, it is important to establish and reflect on career goals. This will help define a preferred practice setting. Reflecting on personal passions and aspirations plays a significant role in this process. Tools like mind mapping can help organize and refine these ideas.

A mind map is a visual tool that connects a central concept to related ideas and details in a non-linear format, resembling a sunburst or spider web [6]. To create a mind map, begin by placing the main goal or topic in the center of a blank page. From there, branch out with related categories such as patient populations, work–life balance, passions, or preferred practice settings. Add details and ideas to each branch as needed. This method can help clear the mind and make room for creativity. This focused exercise can help individuals identify potential job options and chart a clearer career path with other aspects of life addressed.

In addition to self-reflection, networking is a helpful component of the job search. Staying connected through NP groups, professional organizations, and conferences provides access to valuable opportunities. Job boards and platforms like Indeed, Nurse.com, and professional association job centers offer tailored job alerts for real-time updates on openings. Membership in professional organizations such as the American Association of Nurse Practitioners (AANP) provides exclusive resources, including career guidance and networking events like the AANP Job Center [7].

Building relationships with recruiters who specialize in advanced practice nursing is another effective strategy as they can match candidates' skills and preferences with less-publicized opportunities. Personal connections, including former preceptors, mentors, and colleagues, often lead to unadvertised positions aligned with individual career goals.

Checking hospital and practice websites for direct postings further expands the search.

Persistence and a positive outlook are key during this process. Rejections are a natural part of the journey and provide valuable learning opportunities for growth. By combining self-reflection, strategic networking, and practical tools like mind mapping, NPs can approach the job market with a clearer mind and confidence.

2.1.2.1 Crafting the Resume: Essential Components

The key components to an NP's resume include education, clinical experience, certifications, and specific skills such as specialized training. This section will review the essentials as well as ways to ensure the resume will stand out among others. For example, if applying for a women's health position, highlighting any women's health clinical hours with a summary of performed procedures during clinical is helpful. It is important to remember that being a new graduate is not detrimental to a job search. There are clinical hours, research projects, and RN experience to highlight. As a registered nurse, one may be in various leadership roles, and in clinical with a preceptor sets the foundation for a new NP position. While the job market is competitive, strategically including these elements will increase the chances of landing the interview.

Contact Information

When providing contact information on a resume, it is important to use only personal contact details rather than current work or school emails. Using a personal email is recommended because school accounts are often deactivated after graduation that can lead to missed communications. Additionally, including a personal cell phone number and home address ensures that the applicant remains accessible to prospective employers. To further enhance contact accessibility, a link to a professional LinkedIn profile can be helpful. Including a small, professional photograph on the resume also adds a personalized touch, making it easier for potential employers to remember the applicant. If a professional photo is not already available, investing in one for use across resumes, social media, and other professional settings can be highly beneficial [7].

Objective/Summary

An effective resume objective is a concise sentence that summarizes the candidate's career goals and the type of position they seek. A modern objective often highlights relevant experience or achievements in one line, such as, "To obtain a new position at a women's health clinic." Tailoring the objective to each specific job is crucial to capture the attention of the reader and make a strong impact. Alternatively, some may choose to label this section as a "career goal" or "statement of goal."

In the main body of the resume, avoid full sentences and instead use phrases or bullet points, ensuring a consistent format throughout. Employers value clear, succinct information, so checking for grammar and spelling errors is essential. First impressions, even on paper, are impactful and can set a strong foundation. Having a trusted colleague review the document helps ensure accuracy and professionalism [8].

Education, Licensure, and Certifications

In the education section of a resume, it is recommended to list the most recent degree first. For students who have not yet graduated, indicating a "projected graduation date" is acceptable. This section should include academic achieve-ments, detailing degrees earned, institutions attended, and graduation dates, along with any relevant coursework or honors [7]. Additionally, highlight licensure as an NP and list any other relevant certifications, such as Advanced Practice Registered Nurse (APRN) or specialty certifica-tions like Advanced Cardiovascular Life Support (ACLS) or Pediatric Advanced Life Support (PALS), even if obtained prior to graduation.

Clinical Experience

This is where one can shine. Even if one is a new graduate, highlighting the clinical experience during the program will help emphasize the exposure with various patient popula-tions and conditions. For example, if the graduate completed over 200 hours in family medicine, highlighting chronic health problems that were managed in that setting such as hypertension, hyperlipidemia, and diabetes is helpful. Shed light on the accomplishments! For example, if one was able to perform over 100 Pap smears with a preceptor during clin-ical, list this. If one is applying to a dermatology practice and spent a semester with a preceptor in that specialty, put that first on the list so it stands out. This would also be something to mention in the cover letter, highlighting any specific dis-orders or procedures done related to that specialty.

Skills

A well-crafted skills section on an NP resume highlights both clinical and interpersonal abilities. Listing clinical skills can include areas like patient assessment, diagnostic reasoning, and proficiency in procedures such as suturing. Additionally, technical skills such as proficiency with electronic health records (EHR) and familiarity with telemedicine platforms help demonstrate an applicant's ability to work efficiently in a digital healthcare environment [7]. Including soft skills, like effective patient communication, empathy, and teamwork, provides a balanced view of the candidate's abilities. Together, these skills give a holistic view of an NP's readiness to contribute positively to a healthcare organization.

Community Engagement/Service

Including community service and engagement activities on an NP resume highlights a well-rounded commitment to the community and a sense of service beyond clinical responsibilities. Volunteer work, participation in health education initiatives, or involvement in local organizations demonstrate dedication to the well-being of the broader population [9]. These experiences not only reflect a candidate's broader commitment to patient care but also create a personal connection with potential employers by showcasing shared values.

For instance, activities such as organizing community health screenings at local health fairs or leading workshops on preventive health are examples of engagement. Including these experiences on a resume offers insight into the candidate's dedication, compassion, and willingness to go beyond clinical duties to serve the community. These qualities are highly valued in healthcare settings and can set a candidate apart from others. Presenting a more comprehensive and meaningful picture of the professional and personal commitment will stand out.

References

Including professional references on a resume or curriculum vitae (CV) can add credibility and provide potential employers with firsthand insights into an applicant's qualifications.

Listing two references directly on the resume may be beneficial if the individuals are notified each time the resume is submitted. Request permission from each reference before including their name and contact information and inform them each time it is sent to a new organization. While many candidates state that references are "available upon request," listing them can be advantageous if space permits. Each entry should include the reference's name, title, contact information, and a brief description of the relationship to the applicant.

From Resume to Cover Letter

Tailoring the resume to the specific job is important, and seeking guidance from faculty, career resources, or professional organizations can provide further insights into crafting an effective document. A well-crafted resume is a foundational step in the job application process, but it is only part of the equation. The next step is creating a compelling cover letter that complements the resume and provides a more personalized narrative. While the resume highlights qualifications and achievements, the cover letter offers an opportunity to demonstrate enthusiasm for the role and showcase how the candidate aligns with the organization's mission. Together, these documents create an impactful application package (see Appendix 2.A).

Cover Letter: Make a Lasting Impression

A thoughtfully written cover letter serves as a concise and personalized introduction. This complements the resume by highlighting the candidate's qualifications and their connection to the role. It begins with a professional greeting and an engaging introduction that explains why the candidate is an excellent fit for the position. The candidate should research the organization and its mission to demonstrate alignment with the organization's values and goals. For example, referencing how the candidate's commitment to patient-centered care matches the organization's focus on holistic health can create a strong connection.

Expressing enthusiasm and showcasing relevant experience are key to making a memorable impression. If applying for a gastroenterology position, mentioning clinical hours in that specialty and specific procedures performed can illustrate readiness for the role. Additionally, sharing a passion for the field and emphasizing how the candidate's skills fulfill the employer's specific needs reinforces their genuine interest and suitability.

A concise, thoughtful cover letter that ties these elements together sets the stage for further professional engagement and opens doors to networking opportunities (See Appendix 2.B).

Networking Strategies for Success

Building a strong professional network begins during schooling, through connections with clinical preceptors and other healthcare team members. These early relationships often open doors to future job opportunities. Student membership in state NP associations and active participation in meetings are valuable for establishing long-term professional relationships. Additionally, online forums and meet-ups facilitate collaboration and knowledge sharing. Maintaining a professional online presence, particularly on platforms like LinkedIn, is also essential, as potential employers often review social media profiles. NPs should review their digital footprint to ensure that it reflects a professional image aligned with their career aspirations. Leveraging digital platforms for networking and showcasing expertise through online communities, digital portfolios, and optimized LinkedIn profiles can significantly enhance visibility and opportunities within the healthcare industry.

Developing a Professional Identify

Nurse practitioners are encouraged to cultivate a strong and positive professional identity, which serves as the foundation for both career advancement and building patient trust. This identity is shaped through education, clinical experience, personal reflection, and active engagement within the healthcare community. Educational achievements provide the essential skills and knowledge for advanced practice, while diverse clinical experiences demonstrate the refined abilities required to excel in patient care. Affiliations with professional organizations further reinforce a commitment to high standards of care and help establish a positive professional image.

A key aspect of developing this identity is reflective practice, a core component of professional growth. Reflective practice involves regularly assessing personal values, beliefs, and experiences. This ongoing self-assessment helps NPs align their behaviors with professional values and ethical standards. By doing this, NPs can create a consistent and authentic professional identity and demons.

Assignment #1: Job Search Strategy, Resume, and Cover Letter

Goal: To develop a strategic approach to job searching, developing a professional resume, and creating a targeted cover letter to align with desired positions.

Objectives:

1. Analyze various job search resources, to develop a plan tailored to securing a position in a preferred NP specialty.
2. Create a professional, tailored resume that effectively highlights relevant skills, clinical experiences, and qualifications.
3. Compose a targeted cover letter that demonstrates enthusiasm for a potential role and aligns personal strengths with the organization's mission.

Job Search Strategy

Instructions: Create a strategic plan outlining the steps you will take in your job search. Identify your preferred practice settings and discuss how you plan to leverage resources such as professional organizations, online job boards, networking

(continued)

(continued)

events, and personal contacts. Consider how these resources can assist you in locating and securing your ideal role.

Resume Crafting

Goal: To create a detailed and tailored resume that highlights relevant skills and experiences for a specific NP specialty or position.

Instructions: Prepare a comprehensive resume that reflects your qualifications and is tailored to your target NP role. Include sections for contact information, objective or summary statement, education, certifications, clinical experiences, memberships, community engagement, and references. Customize this resume to align with the specific NP specialty you are pursuing.

Cover Letter Writing

Instructions: Draft a cover letter addressing a hypothetical hiring manager for an NP position. Express your enthusiasm for the role and organization, emphasizing strengths, achievements, and alignment with the employer's mission and values. Ensure that your writing is clear and professional and demonstrates an understanding of how your skills meet the employer's needs.

Rubric

Compo-nent	Criteria	Excellent (3)	Proficient (2)	Needs Improvement (1)
Job Search Strategy	Strategic Planning	Outlines a clear, detailed job search plan with multiple resources and preferred settings	Identifies key resources and settings but lacks specific details	Lacks clear plan or identification of resources and settings
	Resource Utilization	Effectively identifies and incorporates multiple networking and job search resources	Identifies some resources; limited networking strategies	Minimal or no use of resources or networking ideas
Resume Crafting	Relevance and Tailoring	Resume is well-tailored to a specific NP specialty and demonstrates relevant experiences	Resume is somewhat tailored but lacks specific customization	Resume lacks relevance or alignment with NP specialty

(continued)

(continued)

Component	Criteria	Excellent (3)	Proficient (2)	Needs Improvement (1)
	Completeness	All relevant sections (contact info, objective, education, etc.) are included and detailed	Most sections are included but lack some depth or detail	Missing essential sections or lacks sufficient detail
Cover Letter Writing	Personalization and Enthusiasm	Cover letter is well-personalized, clear, and reflects strong enthusiasm for the role	Cover letter shows some personalization; enthusiasm is moderate	Lacks personalization, enthusiasm, or is too generic
	Clarity and Professionalism	Writing is professional, clear, and free of errors	Mostly clear and professional; minor errors present	Lacks clarity, professionalism, or contains multiple errors

Assignment #2: Professional Online Presence

Goal: To develop a professional online presence that highlights expertise and supports a positive digital footprint.

Objectives:

1. Evaluate online professional platforms to identify elements that enhance or detract from an NP's professional profile, using specific examples to support recommendations.
2. Design a professional online presence by updating a LinkedIn profile with a professional headshot and engaging content that highlights expertise, achievements, and affiliations.

Instructions: Update your LinkedIn profile with a professional headshot and engaging content that showcases your expertise, achievements, and professional affiliations. Find and participate in one relevant online forum related to NP practice.

Discussion Questions:

1. How can the NP strengthen their online profile? Give two specific examples.

(continued)

(continued)

2. Search internet platforms (Facebook, Instagram, LinkedIn, etc.) for two postings that would *negatively* impact an individual's professional profile. Find two postings that would *positively* impact an individual's professional profile. Explain why you chose these posts.

Assignment #3: Case Scenario Discussion

Goal: To analyze strategies for developing a strong professional identity and online presence.

Objectives:

1. Identify strategies to strengthen his professional identity.
2. Evaluate the potential outcomes of maintaining a strong professional identity.

Instructions: Read the case and answer the questions.

Case:

Olim, an NP just started his first day working in a family practice clinic. His typical schedule is set for

Monday through Friday 7:30 a.m.–4 p.m. After the first year of practice, Olim is thinking of changing clinical practice settings, possibly in a specialty setting. He wants to develop his online presence and strengthen his professional identity.

Answer the following questions:

1. Name and describe two ways Olim can strengthen his professional identity. Be specific, with websites (if applicable) and examples.
2. What would the preferred outcome be for Olim if he maintained a strong professional identity?

Assignment #4: Developing a Professional Bio Assignment

Goal: To create a compelling and professional bio that effectively highlights expertise, accomplishments, and personal attributes.

Objectives:

1. Describe the importance of a professional bio for the NP.
2. Identify the key components of a professional bio.

(continued)

(continued)

3. Develop a professional bio tailored to an NP position.

4. Critically evaluate and revise the professional bio as needed for clarity, professionalism, and impact.

Instructions:

Using the provided guidelines and considering the purpose, audience, and platform, craft a professional bio for an NP position.

Components:

Name and contact information.

Current Role: A brief description of the individual's current position, role, or expertise.

Value: A statement or paragraph highlighting what one can offer to their employer if applicable.

Professional Accomplishments: Brief mention of key achievements, awards, or recognitions.

Personal Attributes: A touch of personal information that adds personality to the bio, such as hometown, family, hobbies, interests, or passions.

Goals and Aspirations: Statements about professional goals, aspirations, or mission.

Professional Expertise/Education: Description of areas of expertise, skills, and knowledge relevant to their profession. Brief mention of relevant educational background, certifications, or qualifications.

Career trajectory if applicable.

Testimonials or Endorsements: Optional inclusion of quotes or endorsements from colleagues, mentors, or clients.

Photo: Professional headshot

Rubric

Criteria	Excellent (4)	Good (3)	Fair (2)	Poor (1)
Components of Professional Bio	Identifies and describes all essential components of a professional bio with detailed explanations	Identifies and describes most essential components of a professional bio with adequate explanations	Identifies some essential components of a professional bio but lacks clarity or detail	Fails to identify essential components of a professional bio
Development of Professional Bio	Develops a well-crafted professional bio with concise and compelling content, demonstrating a strong understanding of target audience and platform	Develops a professional bio with relevant content but may lack some clarity or organization	Develops a basic professional bio with limited detail or relevance to target audience or platform	Fails to develop a professional bio or contains significant errors in content or format

(continued)

(continued)

Criteria	Excellent (4)	Good (3)	Fair (2)	Poor (1)
Professionalism and Personalization	Demonstrates a clear balance of professionalism and personalization, effectively displaying the NP's expertise, accomplishments, and personality	Maintains a good balance of professionalism and personalization, with some aspects effectively showcasing the NP's expertise, accomplishments, and personality	Attempts to balance professionalism and personalization but may lack coherence or effectiveness in showcasing the NP's expertise, accomplishments, and personality	Lacks balance between professionalism and personalization, resulting in an ineffective portrayal of the NP's expertise, accomplishments, and personality

Summary

This chapter provides practical guidance for the transition from NP student to practicing NP, emphasizing certification, job preparation, and professional development. Beginning the job search early and customizing resumes and cover letters for each role demonstrate both professionalism and genuine enthusiasm for specific opportunities. Showcasing relevant skills, accomplishments, and certifications strengthens a candidate's appeal and readiness for the responsibilities of the field. Beyond job-specific skills, maintaining an active professional presence and engaging in organizations are helpful for career growth and networking. These connections offer not only job opportunities but also ongoing support for professional development. Establishing a professional image that reflects ethical standards of nursing contributes to a positive reputation within the community.

References

1. New York State Education Department, Office of the Professions (NYSED). (n.d.). Nurse Practitioners. https://www.op.nysed.gov/professions/nurse-practitioners/how-to-apply (accessed 22 October 2024).
2. American Association of Nurse Practitioners (AANP). (n.d.). Practice Information by State. https://www.aanp.org/practice/practice-information-by-state (accessed 24 October 2024).
3. American Nurses Credentialing Center (ANCC). (n.d.). Certification. https://www.nursingworld.org/ancc/ (accessed 22 October 2024).
4. American Academy of Nurse Practitioners Certification Board (AANPCB). (n.d.). Certification.https://www.aanpcert.org/ (accessed 25 October 2024).

5. Pediatric Nursing Certification Board (PNCB). (2023). Certification Information. https://www.pncb.org (accessed 22 October 2024).

6. Baghestani Tajali, A., Sanatjoo, A., Behzadi, H., and Jamali, H.R. (2023). Use of mind mapping in search process to clarify information needs and improve search satisfaction. *J. Inf. Sci.* 49 (5): 1417–1427. doi: 10.1177/01655515211058041.

7. American Association of Nurse Practitioners. (n.d.). Resume Writing: Tips for Nurses.

8. Mantis, J. (n.d.). A Top-Notch Resume Is Your Gateway to the Job Interview. AANP JobCenter. https://jobcenter.aanp.org/career-advice/a-top-notch-resume-is-your-gateway-to-the-job-interview/116/ (accessed 1 November 2024).

9. Kohler, C. (n.d.). 4 Things You Forgot to Include on Your Resume. AANP JobCenter. https://jobcenter.aanp.org/career-advice/4-things-you-forgot-to-include-on-your-resume/117/ (accessed 1 November 2024).

2.A   Appendix A

Resume Example
[Your Name]
[CityState] | [Phone Number] | [Email Address] | [LinkedIn Profile URL]

Objective

To obtain a position in a women's health clinic where clinical experience and a commitment to patient-centered care can be fully utilized to improve community health outcomes.

Education

Le Moyne College, NY
Master of Science in Family Nurse Practitioner

Anticipated Graduation: May 2025
Le Moyne College, NY
Bachelor of Science in Nursing
Graduated: May 2020
Sigma Theta Tau International Honor Society for Nursing

Clinical Experience

Nurse Practitioner Student
The Women's Health Center at Clinton Family

Preceptor: [Dr. Charlotte Grace]
Jan 2024–Apr 2024

Provided comprehensive obstetrics and gynecology care to immigrant populations facing healthcare access challenges, performing key procedures including Nexplanon insertions.

Nurse Practitioner Student
Comprehensive Breast Care at Rochester General Hospital.

Preceptor: [Dr. Alan Brown NP]
Sept 2023–Dec 2023

Worked alongside the oncology team to deliver patient-centered care for women,
undergoing breast cancer treatment, including treatment monitoring and assessments.

Nurse Practitioner Student
Panorama Pediatric Group

Preceptor: [Genevieve Grace Ramirez NP]
Jun 2023–Aug 2023

Conducted assessments and well-child visits, educating families on growth and vaccination schedules for pediatric patients.

Nurse Practitioner Student
Fairport Baptist Homes

Preceptor: [Dr. Timothy Dell'Anno]
Mar 2023–May 2023

Offered primary care to elderly residents, developing individualized care plans and conducting routine skin assessments.

Nurse Practitioner Student
Lymphoma Clinic at Lipson Cancer Center

Preceptor: [Dr. Peter Moore]
Jan 2023–Mar 2023

Employed telemedicine to provide oncology consultations to adults with lymphoma, enhancing healthcare access for rural patients.

Professional Experience

Registered Nurse

Rochester Regional Health Urgent Care
Jan 2023–Present

Assess and treat patients with acute illnesses in a busy urgent care setting, collaborating with advanced practice providers for effective care delivery.

Created and led a Pediatric Champion initiative to improve pediatric care education among nursing staff.

Registered Nurse
Rochester General Hospital, Pediatric Hematology/Oncology
Jul 2019–Jan 2023

Provided specialized nursing care for pediatric hematology and oncology patients, collaborating with the healthcare team for comprehensive acute care.

Served as charge nurse and mentor for newly hired nurses, supporting family-centered care during critical times.

Registered Nurse
Rochester Regional Health Deployment for COVID-19 Relief
Apr 2020–May 2020

Delivered nursing care to adult patients in a high-demand medical/surgical unit during the COVID-19 pandemic

Patient Care Technician
Rochester Regional Health
Jun 2016–Jul 2019

Actively participated in unit leadership as the patient care technician representative on the unit council.

Certifications

American Heart Association (AHA) Basic Life Support (BLS), AHA Pediatric Emergency Assessment, Recognition, and Stabilization (PEARS)

Association of Pediatric Hematology/Oncology Nurses Chemotherapy/Biotherapy Provider

Professional Memberships

Member, American Association of Nurse Practitioners (AANP)

Member, The Nurse Practitioner Association New York State (The NPA)

Core Competencies/Skills

Clinical skills: Telehealth, diagnostic reasoning, suturing, and EHR proficient

Technical skills: Proficiency with EMR systems, telehealth platforms, and Microsoft Office Suite

Soft skills: Effective patient communication, collaboration, adaptability, and empathy

Community Engagement

8/2023 and 8/2024: NYS Fair Booth. Blood Pressure Screenings.

10/2022 to present: Food Pantry Volunteer

References [give at least 2 references]

1. Ann Tutino-Bean [add contact info)
2. Josephine Devoid Dell'Anno [add contact info]
3. Pesto Wassily Kandinsky [add contact info]

2.B Appendix B

Cover Letter Example
[Your Name]
[Your Address]
[City, State, Zip]
[Email Address]
[Phone Number]
[Date]

Dr. Sylvia Joan CEO (*always name the person*)
[Organization Name]
[Organization Address]
[City
State
Zip]

Dear Dr. Joan:
I am writing to express my enthusiasm for the Nurse Practitioner position at [Organization Name]. With a strong foundation in patient-centered care and a passion for positive health outcomes, I am thrilled at the opportunity to contribute to your team. The mission of [Organization Name] resonates deeply with my commitment to providing compassionate, evidence-based care to diverse patient populations.

With [X years] of experience as a registered nurse and recently obtaining my NP certification, I have developed a skill set that uniquely positions me to excel in this role. My clinical background in [specific area of expertise, e.g., gastroenterology, family practice, pediatrics, etc.] has honed my ability to manage the types of complex patient cases your organization deals with. Additionally, my recent work in an outpatient setting has given me insights into the continuity of care needed to maintain patient health and well-being, especially for those managing chronic conditions.

One of my most fulfilling accomplishments involved [briefly describe a relevant accomplishment or project, e.g., implementing a patient education program or contributing to a protocol]. This experience not only sharpened my clinical skills but reinforced my dedication to initiatives that drive positive health outcomes.

Thank you for considering my application. I am excited about the possibility of contributing to your healthcare team and furthering [Organization Name]'s mission of providing exceptional care.

Sincerely,
(Sign here)
(Printed Name)

Chapter 3

Interview Mastery

Louise Dean-Kelly, PhD, DNS, FNP, RN

School of Nursing, State University of New York Polytechnic Institute, Utica, NY, USA

Practice Manager Perspective
Martha Stevener
Gastroenterology and Hepatology of CNY

Nurse Practitioner: Transition Guide, First Edition. Sara L. Gleasman-DeSimone.
© 2025 John Wiley & Sons, Inc. Published 2025 by John Wiley & Sons, Inc.

Chapter Highlights

Types of Interviews
The five Cs and three Ps of Interviewing
Interview Preparation
Interview Questions
The START Method
The Mock Interview
Post-Interview Strategies
START Worksheet for Behavioral Interview Questions
Mock Interview Grading Rubric
Mock Interview Evaluation Rubric

Chapter Objectives and Mapping to 2021 AACN Essentials

1. Prepare and organize interview materials using evidence-based techniques and understand the health care organization's mission, values, and recent publications. Domain 2: Person-Centered Care. Domain 10: Personal, Professional, and Leadership Development Descriptor

2. Demonstrate the Situation, Task, Action, Result, Tieback/Takeaway (START) method for answering behavioral interview questions by practicing with mock interviews and receiving feedback from peers or mentors. Domain 2: Person-Centered Care. Domain 9: Professionalism Descriptor

3. Evaluate and enhance their interpersonal communication skills by practicing responses to difficult patient interaction questions and demonstrating emotional intelligence during mock interviews. Domain 1: Knowledge for Nursing Practice Descriptor

4. Develop and implement effective post-interview follow-up strategies, including crafting professional thank-you notes or emails and utilizing best practices for post-interview communication. Domain 10: Personal, Professional, and Leadership Development Descriptor:

3.1 Introduction

This chapter will review the types of interviews you may encounter in your search for a position. Emphasis will be placed on the most common types of interviews you will encounter as advanced practice health care professionals. Tips for preparing for and completing the interview process will be discussed. A technique for preparing for the most common types of interview questions will be proposed and explained. The opportunity to practice for your interview will be explained, and an assignment at the completion of the chapter material will assist you in the development of the skills needed to have a successful interview.

"As a practice manager who has been on the hiring end of Nurse Practitioners for over 30 years in this area, the guidelines our practice tends to use in choosing a viable candidate are more based on a personality basis during the interview day itself. We know and trust the rigorous educational program the candidate has gone through in obtaining their master's in nursing to obtain their certification and license. So, we are more looking for how they interact an interpersonal relationship with our patients, colleagues, and support staff. We emphasize instinct and observation during real-world scenarios. Each would have to trust their own instincts in recognizing these features. Tools we use upon interview are bringing them into our endoscopy unit to meet our physicians while they scope – how do they react when they are in the rooms. Or perhaps, we would have them shadow an existing /physician assistant to gauge their responsiveness and adaptability. Red flags during the interview process include candidates who show malcontent, express limitations on schedules with patients right away, or if too reserved."

3.2   What Is an Interview?

An interview in its simplest form is a meeting where two or more people meet to ask and answer questions [1]. For advanced health professionals, a job interview is a structured conversation or meeting between two or more participants used to assess potential employees' qualifications, compatibilities, and character for a particular position. The interviewer is trying to determine whether you are suitable for the position you are seeking; do you have the skill set and experience required for the position; and does the information on your resume matches with your described skill set and experience.

There are many different types of interviews one may participate in during their job search. Box 1 identifies a number of different types of interviews one may encounter during their job search process.

3.2.1   Types of Interviews

Although there are many different types of interviews (see Box 1), the most common you will encounter are **Behavioral, Structured,** and **In Person**. If you are applying for a position at a great distance from your home, your first interview may be **Virtual** or **Online** and some

Box 1 Types of interviews [2, 3]

Screening: This is a short interview to help the hiring person determine whether the potential candidate meets the basic requirements for the position.

Phone: This is often the first of multiple interviews to determine whether a candidate fits with the position and the organization's goals and needs. These are typically screening interviews.

Behavioral: This type of interview gathers information about a candidate's current performance by asking questions about previous situations. Interviewees can use a situation, behavior, and outcome (SBO) method, formerly known as the **S**ituation-**T**ask-**A**ction-**R**esult (STAR) or Situation, Task, Action, Result, Tieback/Takeaway) START method to answer questions. **This is most likely the type of interview you will experience.**

Traditional: This is an in-person interview at the place of potential employment in an office.

Group: This type of interview includes a single interviewer interviewing multiple candidates at the same time. Not usual for health care professionals

Panel: In this type of interview, one candidate is interviewed by multiple members of a hiring team.

Structured: In this type of interview, all candidates are asked the exact same questions in the exact

(continued)

(continued)

same order and their responses are rated on a predetermined scale

Unstructured: This is a **qualitative** type of interview where data are collected by asking any number of questions on a topic in no particular order.

Informal: This is an interview that takes place outside of the office or organizational setting, in a casual setting like at lunch or coffee.

Video/Virtual/Online: These are remote interviews that take place over the Internet either with specialized interview software or software platforms like Zoom or Skype.

Stress: This is an interview where the candidate is presented with a stressful situation and asked to manage it on the spot. The goal is to see how the candidate reacts to this stressful situation.

Case: This occurs when the candidate is asked to solve a specific case (usually in business interviews). These can also be used with health professionals to see how they would handle a specific case as it develops.

Working: This is where the candidate is actually put in the work situation to see how they perform.

organizations may want you get involved in a **Working** interview although it will probably not be your first interview. In-person interviews are self-explanatory; they occur at the site of potential employment in person. **Structured** interviews are ones where the interviewer, or interviewers, asks predetermined questions to all candidates so that they can compare different candidates' responses to specific situations.

You will most probably experience a **Behavioral Interview**. In this type of interview, you are generally asked to explain how you responded to specific situations encountered in the past, or how you used your skills to solve a problem in the workplace. This type of question has been found to provide the interviewer with the most accurate information about how you actually react to certain situations. Evidence shows that when asked how they will react to a situation in the future, candidates typically respond with the best practices known rather than how they, as an individual, will react to the situation. They put themselves in the best possible light in response to the question. If one wants to learn how a person actually responds to a situation, they will ask how you responded to a specific situation, or the type of situation you experienced, in the past. While your response may not be totally accurate, as it is a past experience and you are recalling a memory, research has shown that the interviewer is more likely to obtain a clearer picture of how you actually respond to asked situations [4–6].

3.2.1.1 The Five Cs of Interviewing

Acronyms with the five Cs are popular in many situations to describe professionals and the attributes that professionals endeavor to attain. Think of the original five Cs for nursing–Compassion, Competence, Confidence, Conscience, and Commitment. The original five Cs for nursing were developed by Roach (1993) [7] and were expanded to eight Cs in 1998 by Pusari et al. They added Courage, Culture, and Communication [8]. There are also five Cs identified as important for interviewing: Competency, Character, Communication Skills, Culture Fit, and Career Direction [9]. Note, some of the "Cs" (competency, culture, and communication) are the same for nursing and interviewing. **Competenc**y refers to the technical skills that enable you to perform the required activities of an advanced practice nurse (NP). **Character** is sometimes referred to as one's work attitude. I believe one could make the case that nursing's Compassion, Conscience, and Commitment Cs equate to the Character of the interviewing Cs. Interviewers sometimes attempt to ascertain one's character by asking why you left previous positions. **Communication skills** are important to all positions. As an advanced practice nurse (NP), you will have developed many positive communication skills. The interviewer will be exploring how well you communicate by asking open-ended questions that require you to elaborate on your thoughts, as well as direct questions that determine how sharp you are in answering questions. **Culture Fit** refers to how well your professional beliefs align with those of your present position, the new position you are applying for, as well as the mission and goals of the organization you are applying to. Asking you how you like or dislike your previous employment organization may be explored, as well as what it is about the position you are seeking that fits with your professional beliefs. This may also be reflective of your Commitment (one of nursing five Cs) to your previous position and hopefully what your commitment might be toward the position you are seeking. The interviewer may seek information about your **Career Direction** during the interview by asking you to explain how this position will continue to move your career in the direction you have explained.

In addition to reviewing the **five "Cs"** of interviewing, you should focus on three items that are essential to a successful interview: **Preparation, Practice, and Positivity**—the **three Ps** of interviews. Preparing extensively around practice and positivity will help you give an edge over other candidates and increase your chances of getting hired [10].

3.3 Preparation for Interview

Preparation for the interview is the most important aspect of the interview.

> **Reading a job description**: There are four main items you should pay close attention to when reading the job description. What **experience** is required for the position, what **skills** are needed to perform the job, what are the **education** or training requirements of the position, and what are the **values** of the company.

Employers prepare their job descriptions to emphasize the skills, experience, and qualifications that are required for the position. You should read the description closely to determine how closely your skills, experience, and qualifications align with the role. Also note what is said about the company's values, mission, and goals. To help you determine whether your values align with the facility you are applying to, you might review the "about us" section on their webpage or review their social media postings. It might also help check out their reviews on Glassdoor, Hoover.com, LinkedIn,

Facebook, Google News, or other similar sites. You can also learn about these aspects of the facility by talking with present and past employees. When one does not research the organization, and role, it reveals an uninterested candidate. By reviewing websites, talking with people, and knowing the mission, values, and achievements of that organization, you show you as an enthusiastic person interested in working at the facility.

Thoroughly reading the job description may also provide you with keywords to mention during your cover letter and subsequent interviews. Some employers use software (applicant tracking systems [ATS]) to search for specific words to do the first elimination of applicants [11]. Carefully including keywords from the job description including plural words, abbreviations, and numbers may prevent you from being eliminated in this first review of candidates' resumes. You should be careful to use the exact same terms from the job description. For example, if the job description reads "five years experience," use those exact words rather than "5 years experience." Changing the word five to the number 5 may cause the software to reject your application before it is even seen by a real person. Changing wording like this for each application will take more time and effort than sending a generic resume, but it is well worth it in the long run if you obtain the position you are seeking. It will help prevent you from being eliminated from the applicant pool because the software did not find the keywords related to the position.

3.3.1 Patient Population

While reviewing the job description, be sure to pay close attention to the patient population referred to in the description. You want to present yourself as familiar with both the organization and the patient population involved. Be sure you are ready for this role with this patient population. Take the time to learn the most common types of medical/health conditions in this patient population and specialty focus area. For example, while applying to an orthopedic practice, highlight any clinical experience in orthopedics, as well as in nursing. If you are a new graduate, you can highlight specific student clinical experiences in orthopedics. Know the most common types of conditions that are treated in orthopedics and be able to communicate what the evidence-based treatments are for those conditions.

3.3.2   What to Wear

In addition to a careful examination of the job description, it will be helpful to prepare how you will present yourself and how you will answer the questions asked.

You are seeking a professional position and therefore you should dress for a professional position. That means business or business casual attire. If you are not sure which is appropriate, you might even contact the facility to ask what their prescribed attire is for health professionals. In general, you should wear neutral colors. White, beige, black, or navy for the main colors with few if any bright colors [12]. Clothes should be clean, as well as wrinkle- and stain-free. Avoid the colors of red and orange. Hair should be neat, clean, and worn up or back and out of the way. A simple style is acceptable. Jewelry should be kept to a minimum, no loud or large earrings of any kind. Men should generally wear a suit and tie or a sport coat with matching or tan pants and tie. Women can wear a dress with a conservative hemline, with or without a blazer, or a pantsuit. Shoes should be polished, closed toes, with flat or low heels [13–15]. Keeping tattoos covered is also a good idea as some facilities have specific requirements about the type of tattoos that can be seen by patients and guests.

Before the interview, you should avoid any alcohol or substance intake and be sure to arrive early to the interview. It is important to bring all necessary paperwork with you and during the interview, be sure to maintain direct eye contact with those interviewing you.

Remember body language is very important in any communication situation. Pay attention to what your feet and hands are doing during the interview process.

3.3.3 What Are You Looking For

Prepare a list of things that you are looking for in your next job. What is the salary you would like, and what is the actual salary you would accept for this position? Remember your actual salary for the position does not just come from your weekly pay. How many actual workdays are required? Is time allowed for the completion of paperwork and patient communication? Be sure to ask about retirement payments by your employer and whether there is any matching available. How much time off and money is provided for continuing education? Are there productivity incentives included? What are the remote opportunities and/or requirements? While reviewing job descriptions and preparing for your actual interview, be sure to refer back to your list of requirements.

3.3.4 Documents to Bring

Be sure to have copies of your resume as well as personal identification when you arrive at the interview. You should also carry supplies like pens, pencils, and a notebook to jot down questions you might want to ask at the end of the interview as well as important information you may find out during the interview.

3.3.5 Practice

Most people are nervous when contemplating an interview. What will they ask? Will I be able to answer their questions? What if I can't think of anything to say? During your interview, you will be asked general questions as well as questions related to the position you are seeking. Some of the general questions you may be asked are identified in the following section. You should review the questions and have answers ready for the interview. You should be comfortable with your answers but do not try to memorize everything as your responses will not sound sincere. You should be sure to speak in a clear voice, not too loud or soft, and avoid tells and body language that may indicate you are nervous. Practicing a mock interview prior to your actual interview can help you identify, and hopefully rectify, any excessive fidgeting, unusual body language, or speech irregularities that might annoy the interviewer.

3.4   Common Interview Questions

Health professional interviews consist of general questions about what you would do in future situations and how you have dealt with past experiences (behavior-based questions). Your actual preparation for the interview should include talking with others in similar positions to help you determine the most likely questions you will be asked to discuss during the interview.

General questions will include some of the following:

Tell me about yourself? This offers you the opportunity to review your education and experience. You should try to include something outside of work that will set you apart from other candidates for the position. Your passion for a hobby or volunteer activities would be appropriate.

Why are you interested in this position? Describe something you have learned about the institution to show you have researched the facility and position to make sure it aligns with your goals and beliefs.

Why did you leave your last position? Try not to be negative about your last position. Instead, try to identify how this position will provide opportunities for you to further your skills.

What are your professional goals? This is your opportunity to identify how you hope to further your learning, education, and skills about your profession and how your goals align with the organization's vision.

How do you see the future of health care? or the role of the NP in health care? This general question seeks to identify your general beliefs about health care and what your beliefs are about the future direction of the NP role and general health care.

3.4.1 Strengths and Weaknesses

While the following two questions are not actually evidence-based in that they do not ask you to describe how you handled a situation in the past, they do require you to think about yourself and tell the interviewer what you think are your best and worst traits. This is often difficult. Focus on your professional strengths and weaknesses rather than your personal ones. Try to identify your strengths that align with what they are looking for in this position. You should also try to avoid identifying strengths and weaknesses that are common in the health care community such as punctuality and organizational skills as they are skills that are considered required of all roles. You want to identify strengths that set you apart from other candidates for this position.

Perhaps, you are excellent at your time management skills and prioritizing tasks required for situations. You can also identify other skills like empathy or a problem-solving skill that will be useful in the position you are seeking.

Strength

- **Give me an example of your greatest strength and tell me why you think this is your greatest strength?**
  Sample answer: You might identify that your greatest strength is the ability to be empathetic. Empathy helps you see situations from different perspectives and arrive at solutions that are unique for individuals as well as positive for the organization. The ability to arrive at unique solutions for your patient is important for many reasons including our increasingly diverse society. It helps assure more positive outcomes for both individual patients and health care in general.

Weakness

- **Give me an example of your greatest weakness and tell me why you think this is your greatest weakness?**

You need to be honest but do not need to overemphasize what you identified as a weakness. There is no right or wrong answer here, but you need to identify a weakness that shows self-awareness on your part and describes the strategies and active plans you are working on to attempt to rectify the weakness. You must be sincere in your answer. Telling the interviewer you have overcome the weakness is not realistic or believable. Try to identify health care industry's weaknesses rather than your own personal weaknesses. Instead of identifying that you are an emotional stress eater, point out that increasing staff workloads interfere with one's ability to multitask well in high-stress environments. Always try to stress safety and best practices in your responses if possible.

Sample answer: I have difficulty delegating tasks to others to complete. This often proves helpful because I can be sure things are done correctly, safely, and by following established best practice guidelines. But, it can also have a negative effect because as workloads increase, I need to be able to prioritize and assign tasks to the best staff as well as manage my time and everyone's time wisely and efficiently.

3.4.2 Questions About Past Experiences

While interviews may be very different depending on the interviewer, the most common types of questions asked of health professionals during the interview are evidence-based behavioral questions. This type of questioning involves asking a person to recall a particular type of situation and relate how they handled that past situation. It also assists the interviewer in determining whether you had the knowledge to solve the situation using the best evidence available to you at the time [4].

3.4.3 The START Method for Behavioral Questions

A proven method to prepare for behavior-based questions is the Situation-Task-Action-Result (**STAR**) [16–18] or the **START** method [19]. Use this method to organize your stories of past experiences that will answer the most likely questions you will be asked. Your first step is to prepare your stories by reviewing the job description. What types of skills and qualities are important to this specific position (re-read the job description)?

The START stories should be about two minutes in length, with 20% of the time spent describing the Situation and Task (S&T); 60% spent in describing the Action taken (A); and the final 20% describing the Result of your action and how they Tieback or Takeaway to the situation (what you have learned) [20].

The S stands for Situation: You will be asked to describe a situation that demonstrates a skill considered essential to the position you are seeking. "Please describe a situation when you encountered a difficult patient who would not be involved in their care. How did you handle this patient situation?" A short couple of sentences can explain the situation. There is no need for an extensive description.

Situation: "In my previous role as an NP, I had a patient who had had very serious bowel surgery that resulted in the revision of an ileostomy and the resulting abdominal wound that was left open. He refused to eat, drink, or attempt any physical therapy (PT) or occupational therapy (OT), yet claimed he wanted to be a full code?"

T stands for Task: What was the goal you had to attain? If you had to go against the advice of others to attain your goal, describe it here. Just identify one goal that is appropriate for this component of your interview even if you had many. It is not necessary to explain all aspects of the situation, rather explain one small part that involved you. **Here is where you should identify your specific responsibilities during the described situation. The S&T components of your story should occupy about 20% of the time spent describing your answer to the interviewers.**

Task (goal): *"the goal was to get the patient to start to eat and drink to provide him with the opportunity to heal."*

A stands for Action: Describe the different actions taken to attain the goal. Be sure to include specific details that emphasize your part in the completion of the task. It is important to clearly state what **You** did to attain the goals, but it is also important to give credit to others if they were involved. Be sure to use the pronouns "we" as well as "I" as appropriate for the situation you are describing. Giving others the credit they are due reflects on your character. You should allocate about 60% of your time describing this entire incident to the Action component.

Action: *"Many of my actions involved frequent coordination with the other departments involved in his care. I contacted the dietary department to make sure they did a thorough dietary history and preferences for this patient. I made sure the broadest possible dietary options were included in the orders, as well as ordering appetite stimulants to be included in his medication list. I contacted his family and friends to assist in obtaining specific food preferences from outside the hospital when possible. I made sure that either I or another staff member was available to spend a few minutes with him during each meal to encourage him to eat. I made sure that different and favored fluids were offered to the patient at least every 30–60 minutes by the staff."*

R stands for Result: Describe the outcome of your actions. What happened and how did the situation end. What did you accomplish, don't be shy about identifying your accomplishments. Try to include a number of positive results.

Result: *As a result of the actions taken, the patient slowly began to eat and drink. Dietary supplements were needed to attain wound healing, but most IVs were able to be discontinued after three weeks.*

T stands for Takeaway or Tieback: Describe how your actions relate back to the original situation identified. If you can identify something you learned from this situation, be sure to talk about it.

Tieback: *In addition to the patient starting to eat and drink, he also became engaged in his OT and PT activities. He was able to be discharged to a rehabilitation center after three weeks and return home after an additional four weeks in the rehabilitation facility. He gained over 20 pounds.*

Takeaway: *This situation reminded me of how important coordination of care is and how important it is to involve family members in a patient's care.*

3.4.4 Behavioral Questions

After identifying the skills and qualities considered important by the prospective employer, you need to identify examples of situations where these skills are important.

Try to think of many different situations you may encounter in your prospective position. There are general situations that are common to most advanced practice nursing positions. Some examples include:

How would you handle a situation with a difficult coworker/patient/employer?

How would you handle an ethical situation concerning your personal ethics or a patient's health care ethical dilemma?

Then, identify a specific situation that answers this question from your past experience and be prepared to explain the situation using the START method. Having reviewed several different situations and having a planned way to answer behavioral questions asked will ease your nervousness and demonstrate you are an organized professional. Behavioral questions start with phrases such as "please describe a situation when"; "what did you do when you encountered ___"; and "please provide an example of."

When using this method, you should strive to use examples that directly relate to the skills and attributes identified in the job description for you position you are seeking. If you have any confusion about the question being asked, be sure to clarify what is being asked before attempting to answer the question [10]. During the preparation for your interview, you should think of situations that are common to your chosen position and work through the START method of answering the question. This way you will have well-thought-out answers that refer to evidence-based practice in your responses. The following examples of behavioral clinical questions are general and are some of the most frequently asked topics.

Integrity: Tell me about an unethical or unprofessional situation or dishonesty you observed in a colleague and how you handled it.

Sample answer: When I was a student NP, I was in one of my clinicals with other family NPs and family residents. There were about eight of us who entered the room with our preceptor of the day to examine a young teenage girl whose mother brought her to the clinic for irregular periods. She was not sexually active and was about 13 years old. The preceptor did a vaginal exam without speaking to the girl and then proceeded to do a breast exam that appeared painful to the girl. He announced everything was normal and told our group to "do your exams." I was horrified by his exam and attitude toward the girl and her mother. I asked the group if there was anyone who had not done a normal exam and everyone said no; they all had done several normal exams, so I told them to leave. Outside the room, the residents protested that the physician would be angry if we did not follow his orders to do the exam. The other NPs agreed that no further exams were to be done on this young girl. I told them I believed we would have been committing sexual abuse on that girl if we continued with multiple exams. Most residents then agreed. The physician was angry with me, and I told him I did not see how any of us would gain any new information or skills from the exam and how upset the girl and her mother were about the prospects of many more exams being performed. He just walked away angry.

Mistake you made: Please think of a clinical mistake you have made. How did you resolve the problem and what did you learn from your mistake.

> **Sample answer:** In an earlier role as a staff nurse, I once did not ask about a component of a patient's health history. When I realized what I had missed, I returned to the patient to obtain the information and informed my supervisor so that we could figure out how to address any possible implications. I learned the importance of addressing each component of the health history when obtaining a patient's history.

Remember health care has many rules and regulations in general and additional specific ones at most institutions. Be sure to emphasize the steps you took to avoid legal mistakes. This shows not only that you know the rules and regulations and take them seriously in your professional practice and show concern about the legal implications.

> **Failure:** Describe a time when you failed at a task. What did you learn from it?
>
> **Sample answer:** When I was a beginner nursing student, I was not able to do a simple injection. I bounced the needle off the patient twice before my instructor held my hand and pushed the needle into the patient. I realized after this that I was pulling back at the last minute for fear of hurting the patient. I re-read an article on pain and realized that the small amount of pain I would inflict far outweighed the benefit from the medication. I also practiced many times on some fruits and convinced my cousin to allow me to inject just the needle into her before attempting the technique on a real patient. I realized the importance of practice prior

to attempting new techniques and spent many hours in the skills lab prior to attempting any new skill on a patient.

Additional examples of commonly asked questions are listed as follows.

- **Undisclosed information:** Think about a patient you have cared for that did not disclose important information to you. How did you manage this patient's care? and what was the outcome? Emphasize what actions you took to assure a positive outcome for the patient rather than why they did not disclose the information or how you found out about the failure to disclose.
- **Difficult patient:** Some patients take more time than others to provide their care. Tell me about a patient who required a lot of your time. How did you provide this patient with the care they needed while still providing adequate care to your other patients. Be sure to choose patient situations that highlight your coping skills. Give details of the situations and how you handled them. If possible, describe a situation that is similar to what you will experience at the position you are applying for. This will show the interviewer that you are prepared for this specific position.
- **Requesting antibiotics:** Tell me about a situation where a patient was requesting antibiotics for a viral infection and describe what you did. Remember the goal of this question is to identify that you are aware of the general and/or specific evidence-based practice guidelines and to showcase your interpersonal communication skills.
- **Diversity, equity, and inclusion**: Working with people from different backgrounds or cultures can present challenges. Describe a time when differences in backgrounds

made communication or work challenging. How did you handle the situation? This question gives you the opportunity to show your knowledge of the need for different evidence-based practices that depend on the diversity of your patient population.

3.5   Mock Interview—Actual Practice for Interview

Another aspect of preparation for your interview is practicing an interview. Doing a mock interview is a good way to prepare for your interview. Although it is a practice interview, you should take it as seriously as you would for your actual interview. You can consider it as a dress rehearsal for your interview. There are a number of things to keep in mind as you do your mock interview.

3.5.1   Choose Your Interviewer Carefully

You may feel more comfortable having a friend or a family member acting as the interviewer, but they may not provide you with objective information about your performance. Try to have a person who has experience interviewing candidates for positions do your interview or have a health professional colleague do your mock interview.

3.5.2   The Setting for the Mock Interview

Do the interview at your workplace, another office, or something that simulates the environment where you will do your actual interview. Arrive early and bring all the things you will bring to the regular interview. You should make sure to bring a copy of your resume or curriculum vitae

(CV) with you as well as any other information they may have requested. You should also bring a notepad so that you can take notes about your mock interviewer's feedback on your performance. Remember this is a dress rehearsal, so you should dress as you would for the actual interview.

You should have prepared answers to several possible questions but avoid sounding like they are canned responses. The interviewer will be looking to determine whether you are prepared to engage in a conversation with him/her to determine whether you are the best candidate for the position you are seeking.

Start off your interview by stating your name, offering a polite greeting and a firm handshake. You can also offer a thank you for the opportunity to interview. Watch your body language, sit up in the chair, and try not to fidget. Maintain eye contact with the interviewer and smile rather than frown during the interview. Try to demonstrate your cultural competence in your answers to the questions and not inject bias.

In addition to the feedback you will receive from the interviewer, it may be helpful to actually video- or audio-tape the interview so that you can review it yourself. This might help you identify speech patterns that are not helpful to your presentation or movements that might distract the interviewer, in addition to whether your actual answers are clear and concise.

3.6   Post-Interview Strategies/Follow-Up Techniques

What are your next steps: You should be offered the opportunity to ask some of your own questions at the end of the interview. Will there be a second interview? and if so determine the day and time of the interview as well as the type of the interview. Second interviews may involve you making rounds with some of the staff you may work with. Ask about the group of people you would be working with and what your specific duties would be. Find out whether they are willing to talk salary, *etc.*, at this interview or if it would be more appropriate for a second interview. Ask the interviewers where they think the facility is headed in the next five years and the prospects for any long-term commitments. These questions will not only provide you with additional information to help you decide if this is the correct position for you, but it also shows your interest in the position and facility. If a position is offered at this time, which would be unusual, it would be appropriate for you to thank the employer and tell them that you need more time to consider the offer. Be sure to ask about the facility's timeline to hire this position and their deadline for your response, as well as what their next steps are regarding the position.

Before leaving the interview, you should ask the interviewer for their business card. This will assure you have the correct spelling of the interviewer's name, the address, and the e-mail address for your thank you note. You should send a thank you note within 48 hours of your interview. In the thank you note, you should try to address something you had learned, appreciated, discussed, or enjoyed about the interview, the more specific that you can be, the better. You should also remind them of your key qualifications and interest in the position. You can ask about the growth opportunities this position will offer you as it will show your interest in continuing your education and this area.

After the interview, you should think about what you had learned about the position and the employer during the interview. Determine whether this position meets your goals and priorities currently. If the employer will require a second interview, you should prepare for that interview. The second interview often involves your direct supervisor and/or coworkers. The types of questions asked at second interviews are generally more specific to the position you are applying for, and the interviewer will be looking for your clinical management and knowledge of the evidence-based treatment modalities for this position. All the first-interview preparation applies to the second interview as well. During this interview, it is a good idea to talk to potential coworkers to determine what a typical day includes as well as what they think about the challenges and opportunities offered by this position. Identifying specific policies involved with the position is important to ascertain at this time to make sure they align with your goals and beliefs.

If you have not heard from the potential employer after the hiring timeline, you should call or email the interviewer or the human resources to identify your continued interest in the position and to determine what the new timeline might be for this position.

3.6.1 Positivity

Positivity is a state of mind that will help you be successful in the pursuit of your goals. Keep this in mind as you prepare for the interview process and practice. This should be active throughout all the interview preparation, your practice, as well as at and after the interview.

3.6.2 Conclusion

The interview for your new role is somewhat of a mystery that can be understood. It will take time and energy on your part but with a serious effort you can learn how to successfully navigate the interview process and obtain a position that will enhance your future professional career.

3.7 START Worksheet for Behavioral Interview Questions

During a behavioral interview, you will be asked to demonstrate skills by describing a past experience. Use the following worksheet that will help you prepare for your interview using the START method.

Skill—what the interviewer is looking for	Situation and Task—describe the situation you were involved with and ONE specific task you accomplished (about 30 seconds)	Action—describe the action(s) you took to complete the task (no more than 1 minute)	Result and Tieback/Takeaway—what were the results of your actions and how do they relate back to the situation and/or what have you learned from your actions (30 seconds)
Difficult Patient			
Integrity			
Failure			
Undisclosed Information			

Requesting Antibiotics	**Diversity, Equity, and Inclusion**	**Multitasking**	**Problem-Solving**	**Conflict Management**	**Teamwork**	**Leadership**

3.8   Assignment Mock Interview

Goal: To provide NPs with practical experience in preparing for and participating in a job interview in their profession.

Instructions

- Research common interview questions for NPs, focusing on both behavioral and clinical competency questions.
- Prepare responses using the START method for at least five behavioral interview questions.
- Review the health care organization's mission, values, and any recent publications or news relevant to your field of interest.
- Prepare to discuss your clinical experience, skills, and examples of teamwork, problem-solving, and patient care.

Mock Interview

- Pair up with a fellow student or a mentor.
- Schedule a 30-minute session in person or online.
- Conduct a mock interview. Videotape the interview.
- Answer at least 10 interview questions, including a mix of behavioral, clinical, competency, and general questions.
- Use the START method for behavioral questions and provide detailed examples from your clinical experience.

Feedback and Reflection

After the mock interview, ask your interviewer to provide detailed feedback on your performance by completing the evaluation rubric for the interview. Review the video and reflect on the experience, including what went well, areas for improvement, and addressing weaknesses. Incorporate the feedback received from your interviewer. Your instructor will review the provided material, including the tape, the interviewer evaluation rubric, and your reflection, and will utilize the grading rubric to offer you additional feedback.

Grading Rubric for Mock Interview

Component	Needs Work	Just OK	Well Done
Preparedness (20%) Prepared setting for recording. Understanding of job description. mission; values; Had required paperwork. Demonstrate preparation for interview questions.	**(0–13.9 pts)** Generally unprepared; poorly prepared setting for interview; lack of understanding of mission/values/ job description; no CV or resume provided.	**(14–15.9 pts)** Addressed four of five areas although some still need work.	**(16–20 pts)** Addressed all components.

(continued)

Grading Rubric for Mock Interview

Component	Needs Work	Just OK	Well Done
Use of the START Method (30%) Demonstrate the knowledge of the steps of the START method; use the START method while answering behavioral questions. Effective application of the START method in answering behavioral questions.	**(0–20.9 pts)** Lacks understanding of the method, when to apply it, and does not apply it effectively.	**(20–23.9 pts)** Understands the method and applies with most of the behavioral questions.	**(24–30 pts)** Understands the method and applies it effectively in answering behavioral questions.
Communication Skills (20%) Maintain eye contact; speak clearly so that easily heard;	**(0–13.9 pts)** Fails to incorporate at least four communication	**(14–15.9 pts)** Incorporates at least four communication	**(16–20 pts)** Incorporates at least five communication

stay positive; don't blame; be respectful and tactful; smile appropriately. Body language use: effective but not overly expressive gestures while speaking; does not fidget or demonstrate other nervous habits.	skills, overgestures during the interview, and fidgets excessively.	skills; does not over-gesture; and only fidgets occasionally.	skills; uses gestures appropriately and does not fidget.
Professionalism (10%) Choice of the interviewer, professional attire, greet the interviewer with a handshake and vocally; asks for a business card at the end of the interview.	**(0–6.99 pts)** Only incorporates two or fewer of the components.	**(7–7.99 pts)** Incorporates three of four components in the interview process.	**(8–10 pts)** Incorporates all components in the interview process.

(continued)

Grading Rubric for Mock Interview			
Component	Needs Work	Just OK	Well Done
Feedback and Reflection (20%) Address all areas for quality and the depth of reflection on the mock interview experience, including the incorporation of feedback/areas for improvement. Preparation; Use of the START method; Communication skills; Professionalism.	**(0–13.9 pts)** Evaluation includes only two areas and does not provide information about strengths/ weaknesses and ways to improve.	**(14–15.9 pts)** Addresses three areas but provides only fair information about strengths and weaknesses and/or ways to improve.	**(16–20 pts)** Provides thoughtful evaluation of all four areas: identifying strengths/ weaknesses and thoughts about improvement strategies.

Evaluation Rubric for Interview

This rubric is developed to help the person acting as the interviewer give feedback to the student acting as the potential job candidate. Please address all areas with a checkmark and provide constructive criticism and positive comments.

	Needs Work	Just OK	Well Done
Preparedness: Location mimicking actual interview setting desk/chairs, quiet, no interruptions, Demonstrated understanding of the job description, including the mission and values of facility/company Brought resume or CV, notepad, and other papers. Have the recording setup ready. Demonstrated preparation for common interview questions as well as clinical and behavioral questions. **Comments:**			

(continued)

	Needs Work	Just OK	Well Done
Use of STAR method- Effective application of the START method in answering behavioral questions. Demonstrated knowledge of the steps of this method. Used the START method while answering behavioral questions. **Comments:**			
Communication Skills (20%): Maintain eye contact; speak clearly so that easily heard; stay positive; don't blame; be respectful and tactful; smile appropriately. Body language use: effective but not overly expressive gestures while speaking. Does not fidget or demonstrate other nervous habits. **Comments:**			

Professionalism:
Choice of the interviewer.
Professional attire.
Greet the interviewer with a handshake and vocally.
Ask for a business card at the end of the interview.
Comments:

References

1. Interview. Cambridge Oxford Dictionary. https://dictionary.cambridge.org/us/dictionary/english/interview (accessed 21 April 2025).

2. Career Guide (2023). Indeed editorial team. https://www.indeed.com/career-advice/interviewing/major-types-of-job-interview

3. Carter, A. (2003). 5 types of interview and how to prepare. https://www.astoncarter.com/en/insights/articles/5-types-of-interviews-and-how-to-prepare#:~:text=There%20are%20several%20different%20types,panel%20interviews%20and%20informal%20interviews (accessed 21 April 2025).

4. Nisbett, R.E. and Wilson, T.D. (1977). Telling more than we can know: verbal reports on mental processes. *Psychol. Rev.* 84 (3): 231.

5. Oostrom, J.K., Melchers, K.G., Ingold, P.V., and Kleinmann, M. (2016). Why do situational interviews predict performance? Is it saying how you would behave or knowing how you should behave? *J. Bus. Psychol.* 31: 279–291.

6. Latham, G.P. and Saari, L.M. (1984). Do people do what they say? Further studies of the situational interview. *J. Appl. Psychol.* 69: 569–573. https://doi.org/10.1037/0021-9010.69.4.569.

7. Roach, M.S. (1993). *The Human Act of Caring: A Blueprint for the Health Professions.* Ottawa: Canadian Hospital Association Press 163 p.

8. Pusari, N.D. (1998). Eight 'Cs' of caring: a holistic framework for nursing terminally ill patients. *Contemp. Nurse* 7 (3): 156–160. https://doi.org/10.5172/conu.1998.7.3.156.

9. Law, E. (2023). The 5Cs interview skills. linkedin.com Available from https://www.linkedin.com/pulse/5cs-interview-skills-eddie-law-%E5%88%98%E7%94%A8%E9%92%BF/ (accessed 21 April 2025).

10. Archambeau, S. 2023. Preparation, practice, & positivity-learn the 3 P's of interviews. https://www.shellye.opengrowth.com/article/preparation-practice-

positivity-learn-the-three-p-s-of-interviews#:
~:text=In%20order%20to%20succeed%20in,your%20
chances%20of%20getting%20hired (accessed 21 April
2025).

11. James H. (2021) How to pick resume keywords That'll get your
application past the ATS. The Muse. https://www.themuse.
com/advice/a-job-hunters-guide-to-getting-your-
resume-past-the-ats-and-into-human-hands

12. Career Builders (2013) The best and worst Colors to Wear in
a job interview. Harris Interactive. https://press.career
builder.com/

13. Elliot, A.J. and Maier, M.A. (2014). Color psychology: effects of
perceiving color on psychological functioning in humans. *Annu.
Rev. Psychol.* 65: 95–120.

14. Johnson, K.K.P. and Roach-Higgins, M.E. (1987). Dress and
physical attractiveness of women in job interviews. *Clothing
Text. Res. J.* 5: 1–8.

15. Baxromov, U. and Xamroxojayev, B. (2024). Visual, imaginary,
psycho-physiological study and scientific analysis of clothing
colors. *AIP Conf. Proc.* 3045 (1): https://doi-org.sunypoly.idm.
oclc.org/10.1063/5.0198287.

16. Jones, R. and Hameed. F.2024). What is the STAR interview
technique. Airswift.https://www.airswift.com/blog/star-
technique-job-interviews (accessed 21 April 2025).

17. Indeed get to know candidates with the STAR interview
format. https://www.indeed.com/hire/c/info/star-
interview-format?gad_source=1&psafe_param=1&
gclid=EAIaIQobChMIwp-Yz-3lhgMVqGFHAR3Q_
Q2NEAAYASAAEgKwKfD_BwE&aceid=&gclsrc=aw.ds (accessed
21 April 2025).

18. Career Advising & Professional Development. Using the STAR
method for your next behavioral interview. https://capd.
mit.edu/resources/the-star-method-for-behavioral-
interviews/ (accessed 21 April 2025).

19. Apple, J.M., Guerci, J.C., Seligson, N.D., and Curtis, S.D. (2021).
Adding the second T: elevating STAR to START for behavioral

interviewing. *Am. J. Health Syst. Pharm.* 78 (1): 18–21. https://doi.org/10.1093/ajhp/zxaa356.
20. Society for Human Resources Management (2016). A guide to conducting behavioral interviews with early career job candidates. https://cassstaffing.org/wp-content/uploads/Behavioral_Interviewing_Guide_for_Early_Career_Candidates_Article.pdf (accessed 21 April 2025).

Chapter 4

Understanding Contracts of Employment

Cynthia Grabski
DNS, FNP-BC
School of Nursing, State University of New York Polytechnic Institute, Utica, NY, USA

Expert Insights: Tips for Successful Negotiation
Virginia Cronin, PhD, FNP-BC
Nascentia Health, Syracuse, NY, USA

Nurse Practitioner: Transition Guide, First Edition. Sara L. Gleasman-DeSimone.
© 2025 John Wiley & Sons, Inc. Published 2025 by John Wiley & Sons, Inc.

Chapter Highlights

Contract Elements
Key Clauses
Employment Types
Compensation
Legal Considerations
Contract Negotiation
Scope of Practice

4.1 Introduction

Starting a new career as a nurse practitioner (NP) is an exciting milestone, but it also comes with new challenges, such as understanding employment contracts. For many NPs, this may be their first encounter with a contract that defines job duties, rights, responsibilities, and compensation. It is easy to feel overwhelmed by the legal language and fine print, especially when it all seems so unfamiliar. This chapter aims to clarify those complexities by breaking down the different types of contracts and explaining common terms. Practical tips for negotiating the best deal will be provided to help NPs approach this process with confidence and clarity. This chapter follows Nancy, a newly graduated NP, as she navigates her first contract. Nancy has been offered a position as a primary care provider. With these objectives in mind, let's follow Nancy as she applies her previous classroom knowledge to this real-world situation.

Nancy, a new NP, has been offered her first position as a primary care provider in a private practice. Nancy knows in

---

Objectives with and Mapping to 2021 AACN Masters Essentials

1. Identify different types of employment contracts for NPs. Domain 1: Knowledge for Nursing Practice
2. Describe the key clauses commonly found in NP employment contracts. Domain 6: Health Policy for Advocacy in Health Care
3. Explain how state-specific Nurse Practice Acts (NPAs) influence contract terms and conditions. Domain 4: Scholarship for the Nursing Discipline
4. Outline strategies for negotiating employment contract terms. Domain 7: Interprofessional Partnerships

---

addition to legal counsel, there are several steps she can take to thoroughly review and understand the document before making a commitment.

4.1.1 Contracts

A contract is a legally enforceable agreement between parties that creates mutual obligations [1]. A legally binding contract requires four key elements: mutual assent, adequate consideration, capacity, and legality. Mutual assent is an offer and acceptance of the offer. Adequate consideration means that each party must receive something of value in exchange. Capacity refers to the mental ability of the parties to understand the terms and consequences of the contract. Legality is the contract's purpose that must be lawful.

Contracts can be governed by three types of law: (1) statutory law, which is established by legislation; (2) common law, which is derived from judicial rulings and interpretations; and (3) private law, which includes the specific terms agreed upon by the parties. Employment contracts are legally binding, and misunderstandings can lead to a breach of contract, potentially resulting in legal action or termination.

Nancy recalls that employment contracts are a type of contract and all elements must be understood by all parties entering into the agreement. In her studies, she learned that contracts need to clearly define the duties to be performed. A mutual agreement and the type of compensation can be expected for the services rendered. Nancy is being offered an employee salary with benefits.

4.1.1.1 Employment Types

The employment contract should clearly specify whether the NP will be an employee of the practice or an independent contractor. An NP who is classified as an employee typically receives a salary with the potential for bonuses. Benefits such as health insurance, dental coverage, malpractice insurance, vacation days, and others are usually included, although the percentage of cost shared between the employer and employee may vary. Additionally the employer withholds local, state, and federal taxes from the employee's pay.

In contrast, independent contractors are only compensated for the services they provide. Typically, these positions do not offer additional benefits, and as an independent contractor, the NP is responsible for paying all personal taxes and securing malpractice insurance [1]. If the NP is an independent contractor, the employment contract should clearly specify who is responsible for covering expenses, such as equipment, staff support, supplies, malpractice insurance, and continuing education. It should also indicate whether these costs will be deducted from the NP's salary and who will bear the upfront costs—the employer or the contractor [1]. Understanding the type of employment is only the first step. Key contract terms and elements every NP should be aware of will be discussed in the following section.

4.1.1.2   Boilerplate Language

"Boilerplate language" refers to the standard legal clauses that are commonly included in most contracts. These clauses cover routine legal matters such as how disputes will be handled (arbitration or mediation), confidentiality requirements, whether a jury trial is waived, and who can take over the contract if needed [1]. Both parties must review these standard provisions with an attorney to ensure full understanding and agreement before signing. While understanding these standard legal provisions is important, NPs should also pay close attention to the specific duties and expectations outlined in the contract, which directly impact their day-to-day responsibilities.

4.1.1.3   Duties, Responsibilities, and Expectations

NPs operate under a defined scope of practice governed by the NPA and state laws, as established by state boards of nursing or medical boards. During the review of an employment contract, it is essential that these documents are available to confirm that the contract does not include responsibilities that exceed the scope of practice as defined by the NPA and state laws [2]. It is also important to consider that requirements for physician supervision and collaboration vary from state to state, so the NP should ensure that all parties agree to the terms of supervision and collaboration before signing.

The contract must also state when the NP is expected to assume full responsibilities. The orientation process should be clearly defined, including the type of training provided, whether electronic medical record (EMR) system training is included, who will oversee the orientation, and the duration of the orientation period.

The contract should clearly specify the type of diagnostic codes and the level of patient complexity that the NP will be expected to manage, as well as the time allotted per patient and the expected daily patient volume. A reasonable cap of 15–20 patients per day after an orientation phase is suggested, depending on the workday length and setting. Additionally, the contract should clarify whether there is a limit on the total patient panel and whether the NP will manage patients independently or in collaboration with a physician.

Specifics such as daily work hours and the number of workdays per week should be explicitly stated. If on-call duties are required, the details of the call schedule and compensation should also be clearly outlined. The contract should specify the type of support staff that will be available, such as a scribe, secretary, or telephone triage nurse. It should also include provisions for the work environment, detailing whether the NP will have access to a private office and exam rooms or if these spaces will be shared with other providers. Finally, the contract should specify the term of employment, including both the start and end dates.

4.1.1.4 Extended Role Expectations

Is there an extended role expectation associated with the position? For example, an extended role might be specialized skills not typically associated with the role of the office-based NP, such as colposcopy training, botulinum toxin injections, or other procedures [3]. This can be interpreted broadly, so it is important to clearly define these expectations. The extended role goes beyond the previously discussed job description and specifies additional skills required to perform the job.

Several considerations should be reviewed to ensure mutual understanding of the terms related to extended role expectations. These include a thorough review of the NPA guidelines, the state NPA, liability coverage, a specific time-frame for initiating the procedure, educational preparation, policy development, and opportunities for clinical practice. The employment contract should clearly outline how the addition of these skills will be compensated for. Another area to consider is the employer's involvement in community outreach programs and the expectations for employee participation. Any expectations for employee involvement should be discussed and clearly defined in the employment contract. Elements such as the frequency of participation, location, and hours of commitment should be included, along with the specific duties to be performed. For example, will the NP be expected to develop community programs or provide medical care at community or school events? [3].

As Nancy reviews the contract, she wonders what the orientation process is like and how long it would be. She wonders if she is going to be trained in in-office procedures and/or need to round at the hospital. As Nancy reviews the compensation section of her contract, she notes that her base salary seems reasonable but isn't sure whether it reflects her full value as a newly credentialed NP and any additional provided services.

4.1.1.5   Compensation and Benefits

Understanding the full scope of compensation and benefits is essential for NPs to ensure that the contract aligns with their professional and personal needs. A comprehensive compensation package goes beyond just the annual salary and should encompass all aspects of financial and non-financial rewards offered by the employer. Properly evaluating these elements is key for NPs to make informed decisions about their career opportunities and financial well-being.

Salary and Bonus Structure

The foundation of any compensation package is the base salary, which should be clearly defined in the contract [2]. The base salary refers to the guaranteed annual income that an NP will receive. It is important for NPs to understand whether their salary is fixed or determined by relative value units (RVUs), which are based on the volume and complexity of services provided.

To assess the value of the position, NPs should consider the practice's charges per patient visit and their expected patient load. When assessing compensation, NPs should account for practice overhead, insurance costs, and expected patient load to ensure that the salary is appropriate for the position. Private practices usually aim for a profit margin of 15–20%, which can help estimate an NP's value to the practice. If an NP's compensation expectations exceed what the practice can afford, based on these calculations, it may pose challenges for the employer to justify the hire [4].

Additionally, NPs can inquire about the availability of a bonus structure. Bonuses may be awarded based on performance metrics such as patient volume, quality of care, or other key performance indicators set by the employer [2]. The contract should also clearly outline the terms of the pay schedule—whether payments are made weekly, bi-monthly, or monthly. NPs should be cautious of contracts where the salary is based on what is collected rather than what is billed, as they have no control over the employer's collection practices.

Health and Wellness Benefits

Health and wellness benefits are a significant component of the overall compensation package and can greatly influence job satisfaction and financial security. These benefits typically include health insurance, dental coverage, and vision plans. NPs should review the cost-sharing details between the employer and employee, such as premium contributions, co-pays, and out-of-pocket expenses. It is also important to consider whether the employer offers additional wellness benefits, such as gym memberships, mental health support, or health savings accounts (HSAs).

Retirement Plans and Insurance Coverage

Retirement plans, such as 401(k) or 403(b) options, should be thoroughly evaluated to understand the employer's contribution, vesting schedule, and available investment options. NPs should also inquire about life insurance and disability benefits, including the level of coverage provided and any options to purchase additional coverage at a group rate. These benefits are essential for long-term financial planning and security, especially in the event of unforeseen circumstances.

Paid Time Off

Paid time off (PTO) policies should be clearly outlined in the contract, including vacation days, sick leave, and personal time off. NPs should check whether different types of leave are allocated separately or combined into a single

PTO bank. If one is transitioning from a registered nurse (RN) role, maintaining current vacation and personal time might be a priority. First, confirm the total amount of vacation or PTO offered annually, ensuring that it aligns with or exceeds what one has been accustomed to as an RN. Many full-time NP contracts offer between two and four weeks of vacation, so it's important to verify whether this time is accrued throughout the year or provided upfront. Look for clear distinctions between vacation, sick days, and personal time, and ensure that one is not moving backward in terms of the flexibility one previously had.

Be sure to understand whether unused vacation or personal time can be carried over to the next year, or if there is a "use-it-or-lose-it" policy in place. Finally, review how the process for requesting time off works, and whether there are any restrictions or blackout periods when vacation requests may not be granted. By carefully reviewing PTO, one can ensure that the work–life balance is protected.

Continuing Education

In addition to vacation and personal time, continuing education days and reimbursement for professional development activities are important aspects of the compensation package. NPs will need hours in continuing education to renew their national certification [2]. Look for specific details about the amount of paid continuing medical education (CME) time provided, ensuring that it is separate from the PTO. Additionally, consider whether unused CME time or funds can roll over to the next year or if they are "use-it-or-lose-it" provisions. Sometimes, CME funds can be used toward certification renewal or Drug Enforcement Administration (DEA) registration fees. Understanding these details will ensure that you are well supported in maintaining your certification as well as professional development.

Relocation and Additional Benefits

For NPs relocating for a new position, the employment contract should specify any relocation assistance, such as moving expenses, temporary housing, or travel reimbursement. Other benefits to consider include malpractice insurance coverage, legal support for contract negotiations, and additional perks, such as sign-on bonuses, loan repayment programs, or flexible work arrangements. NPs should confirm whether the employer provides financial support for certification, DEA renewals, or membership dues [2].

Nancy recalls a conversation with her mentor, who emphasized the importance of understanding not just the salary itself but also the total compensation package. In addition to salary, the contract offers bonuses based on patient volume and performance metrics like patient satisfaction. Nancy wonders how these bonuses will be calculated and whether they will truly reflect the complexity of the cases she handles. If she is expected to round the hospital before or after office hours, she asks how this is included in the compensation package. If Nancy is on call three days a week in the evening, is that extra or included in the salary.

4.1.1.6 Contract Clauses

Contract clauses are special provisions included in employment agreements to address specific details that go beyond the standard boilerplate language. Once an employment contract is signed, it is considered accepted "as is" unless specific clauses have been added beforehand. This means that if a particular detail is not explicitly stated in the contract, neither party is obligated to agree to changes after the fact. These clauses are essential for tailoring the contract to the unique needs of both the employer and the NP. They provide clarity on important issues and help prevent misunderstandings in the future. Common types of contract clauses include termination terms, restrictive covenants, and tail coverage for malpractice. Each of these clauses serves a specific purpose in defining the rights and responsibilities of the parties involved and should be carefully reviewed to ensure that they align with the professional and legal expectations of the NP role.

Termination Clause

The termination clause in an employment contract outlines the conditions under which the employment relationship may be ended by either party. It is essential that this clause provides clear information about whether termination can occur with or without cause, and it should include explicit examples of actions or inactions that could lead to termination. The contract should specify whether the employer has the right to terminate the agreement without providing a reason, known as termination without cause.

Additionally, the clause should detail the notice period required before termination takes effect and any obligations during this timeframe. It should also address the process for paying out any salary, bonuses, and benefits earned up to the termination date. This ensures that both parties are aware of their rights and obligations if the employment relationship ends [5].

Nancy sees that she needs to give a 12-month notice to end this new contract. If she is having a hard time and wants to switch jobs after 6 months, giving a 12-month notice does not seem reasonable.

Restrictive Covenant

A restrictive covenant, commonly referred to as a non-compete clause, is a contractual provision designed to protect the financial interests of the employer by limiting the NP's ability to work for competing practices during and after employment. These clauses typically serve two primary purposes: they prevent the NP from working for another employer while still employed by the current practice (often referred to as moonlighting) and impose geographic restrictions on where the NP can practice after leaving the job. This geographic limitation is meant to prevent the NP from providing services within a specific area that could compete with the former employer.

NPs should be aware of the state laws governing restrictive covenants, as not all states permit them. For instance, in 2024, the Federal Trade Commission (FTC) issued a Final Rule that sought to invalidate non-compete clauses in standard employment agreements. However, this rule was struck down by the United States District Court for the Northern District of Texas, citing that the FTC had exceeded its authority [6].

As of July 2022, 12 states have prohibited restrictive covenants by statute, while the remaining states and territories allow them either by common law or statute [7]. In most employment contract negotiations, NPs may find these clauses to be non-negotiable. It is important to understand the specific regulations regarding geographic restrictions and timeframes in their state before signing an agreement [7].

Non-solicitation and Evergreen Clauses

A non-solicitation provision is often included alongside a restrictive covenant in employment contracts [3]. This provision prohibits an NP from encouraging or persuading patients to leave the current practice and follow them to a new one after their employment has ended. However, if patients independently choose to seek care from the NP at their new practice, without any solicitation, this is considered a voluntary act and does not constitute a breach of contract. It is important for the NP to ensure that any communication with their patient panel during the transition period cannot be interpreted as an attempt to solicit those patients.

An evergreen clause, on the other hand, automatically renews the employment contract on a predetermined date unless one party provides notice to terminate or renegotiate. The advantage of this clause is that it eliminates the need to renegotiate a contract that both parties find satisfactory. However, the downside is that it may limit the NP's ability to make desired changes to the contract, such as negotiating for a raise, adjusting their schedule, or modifying job responsibilities. This lack of flexibility can be a disadvantage if the NP's needs or career goals change over time.

Liquidation Clause

A liquidation clause, also known as a liquidated damages clause, outlines the financial consequences an employee may face for terminating the contract before the agreed-upon end date [3]. This clause is particularly important in employment agreements for NPs, as it establishes a predetermined penalty or "cost" for early termination. The purpose of a liquidation clause is to compensate the employer for potential losses resulting from the NP's premature departure, such as recruiting and training expenses for a replacement, service disruptions, or lost revenue. This can have significant financial and professional repercussions if the NP decides to leave the position early. Unreasonably high penalties may be deemed unenforceable in court, as they could be considered punitive rather than compensatory. According to the American Association of Nurse Practitioners (AANP), it is essential for NPs to be fully aware of all contract terms, including liquidation clauses, to protect their professional and financial interests [4].

Performance Review

A performance review clause provides the NP with structured feedback and sets clear expectations. NPs should ensure that performance criteria, such as patient load, satisfaction, and adherence to guidelines, are defined clearly in the contract. Additionally, the clause should specify the frequency and format of performance reviews. Will they occur annually, biannually, or quarterly? Will they include self-assessments, peer reviews, or patient feedback? Clarifying these details in advance helps NPs prepare and address areas for improvement proactively. A transparent and well-defined performance review process is essential for NPs to understand how their contributions are valued and to advocate for their professional development [3].

Nancy sees that she will get an initial performance review at six months, then yearly with the potential for 5% raises. Nancy feels good that she will have the opportunity to address areas for improvement.

Liability Coverage

Extended liability coverage, or "tail coverage," is an essential provision in an employment contract for NPs because it provides continued protection against malpractice claims that may arise after the NP has left the practice [8]. Without this coverage, NPs could be personally liable for any claims made for incidents that occurred during their employment but are reported after their departure. The specifics of this clause should include who is responsible for paying the premiums, whether it is the employer or the NP, as well as the duration of the coverage. Typically, tail coverage can be purchased for varying timeframes, such as 1, 3, or even 10 years, depending on the terms negotiated. Negotiating the inclusion of extended liability coverage in the employment contract is crucial, particularly for NPs who are transitioning to a new job or leaving the practice altogether. It is important to confirm whether the employer will cover the cost of tail coverage or whether the NP will be required to bear this expense.

Financial and Legal Considerations

The cost of tail coverage can be significant, often amounting to several thousand dollars, which can be a financial burden if not planned for. NPs should consult with an attorney experienced in health care law to ensure that coverage limits are adequate and that there are no gaps in protection that could expose the NP to legal and financial risks. According to the AANP, understanding the details of malpractice insurance, including tail coverage, is a key factor in safeguarding one's professional practice and financial security [9].

Nancy nurse believes she has identified all the additional clauses to be included in her contract. She is positive that a well-crafted employment contract will be drafted. Nancy believes she can meet the employment contract obligations and she will not be at risk for breach of contract during her tenure in the practice.

4.1.1.7 Breach of Contract

A breach of contract occurs when one of the parties involved in an agreement fails to fulfill their obligations as outlined in the contract [3]. This failure can take several forms, including not performing a duty at all, performing it inadequately, or violating specific terms of the agreement. For NPs, a breach could involve issues such as not adhering to the scope of practice, failing to meet productivity expectations, or not maintaining required licensure and certifications. Conversely, an employer could breach the contract by not providing agreed-upon compensation, benefits, or a safe working environment.

When a breach occurs, the non-breaching party has the right to take legal action to seek remedies, which may include financial compensation, specific performance (requiring the breaching party to fulfill their obligations), or termination of the contract without penalty. The type of remedy pursued often depends on the nature and severity of the breach, as well as the specific terms outlined in the contract. It is important for NPs to understand the conditions that constitute a breach and the potential consequences, as a breach can not only lead to financial losses but also damage professional relationships and reputations [3].

4.1.1.8 Recognizing Red Flags

When reviewing an NP contract, it is crucial to identify terms that could negatively affect both professional and personal life. One red flag is an excessively long notice period, such as a 12-month requirement for terminating employment, which can limit the NP's ability to pursue other opportunities. Noncompete clauses that restrict practice within a specific geographic area or specialty after leaving the organization can also have significant consequences for future career options. Compensation structures based on productivity bonuses should be scrutinized to ensure that expectations are clear, realistic, and achievable. For example, a reasonable salary might seem fair, but if the NP is required to be on call every weekend and one evening a week without any additional compensation, the contract may not be as favorable as it first appears. Vague job descriptions or unclear on-call duties can lead to role confusion and potential burnout. Additionally, a lack of support for continuing education or professional development may suggest that the organization is not fully committed to the NP's growth and long-term success. Clauses that allow the employer to unilaterally alter contract terms or demand repayment of benefits or bonuses if the NP leaves before a certain period should also be approached with caution. Addressing these issues before signing is vital to ensure that the contract supports both the NP's professional goals and personal well-being.

As Nancy digs deeper into her first employment contract, she begins to apply the knowledge she acquired as well as any legal counsel. Her first step was to assess the type of employment being offered—whether she will be classified as an employee or an independent contractor. During her initial meeting with the potential employer, Nancy asks specific questions about her classification and the associated benefits, such as health insurance and retirement plans. She recalls the importance of understanding these distinctions because they significantly impact not only her take-home pay but also her tax responsibilities and access to benefits. Nancy uses this information to negotiate a clear and fair compensation package that aligns with her professional goals and personal needs. As the negotiation progresses, she confidently discusses the inclusion of a termination clause that provides her with sufficient notice and safeguards her from unexpected job loss, demonstrating her thorough understanding of the contractual elements.

> "Let us never negotiate out of fear. But let us never fear to negotiate"—John F Kennedy

Expert Insights: Tips for Successful Negotiation
By Virginia Cronin, PhD, FNP-BC

Negotiating a provider contract can be daunting, but understanding the psychology behind the process can improve your negotiation skills. Having taught and precepted new NPs for over 20 years, my best advice to students entering the health care marketplace is to:

1. **Know your potential employer:**
   Is the company for-profit or not-for-profit? What is the mission or vision of the organization? What population do they serve? A small practice or a rural practice that provides care for predominantly low-income or underserved populations may not have the ability to offer a wide salary range compared to a large, multistate health system.

2. **Have a realistic understanding of what you have to offer an employer as a novice NP:**
   As a new graduate, your advanced practice clinical experience is limited to what you've done in your preceptorship, which may put you at a disadvantage. You'll likely be offered a starting salary commensurate with your experience. However, your first job will not likely be your last. Once you gain practice experience, you have more leverage to push back on salary negotiations. That being said, how can you set yourself apart

from other NPs vying for a position? Perhaps you may have completed more than the required clinical hours for your program to gain additional exposure to medicine. Maybe you have completed a clinical internship with the company. If you have significant nursing experience, how do you use that experience to help position you for a job. The hiring manager for a cardiology group would likely be more interested in a new NP with five years of nursing experience on a cardiac floor or Critical Care Unit (CCU) than a new NP with five years experience in Med-Surge.

3. **Have a basic understanding of market opportunities that exist to bolster your negotiation strategies:**
   Look at job boards like Monster, Indeed, and ZipRecruiter to see what NPs' salary ranges are being offered in your area so that you have a starting point for negotiating. If there are limited NP opportunities in your community and a lot of NP grads, the employer has an advantage, and you may have not had much room to negotiate the offer. Conversely, if there are few NPs and many job opportunities, then you have the upper hand in negotiating.

4. **Understand the negotiables:**
   It's not just your salary that you want to negotiate. You also have the opportunity to negotiate "reimbursables"— the fees associated with keeping your practice current. These fees can include licensing fees, malpractice insurance, and continuing education fees.

   If time is more important to you than money, then you may want to negotiate more vacation time or flex time once a week.

5. **Be confident and take good notes:**
   The best way to bolster confidence is to do your research and interview for multiple positions. In my opinion, it's better to have multiple offers to consider than just one. The more offers you have, the stronger your negotiating position. With multiple offers, you may be able to increase your salary, compensation for reimbursables, or benefits, by playing one potential employer's offer against another. The worst that can happen in a negotiation is that the employer holds firm to an offer.

   The goal of negotiating is to arrive at a mutually agreeable offer. Don't be pressured into making a quick decision. Always ask for a day or two to think about the offer and the total compensation package. If you have further questions, don't be afraid to ask them. Understand that compromise is mutual—be flexible, but be prepared to graciously walk away if the offer is low or too rigid. If you are satisfied with the offer, take it!

Assignment #1:   Employment Contract Evaluation for NPs

Goal:

To enable students to critically evaluate employment contracts by understanding the legal and professional implications specific to NPs.

(continued)

(continued)

Learning Objectives:

Identify practices or legal services available for employment contract reviews specific to NPs.

1. Analyze the non-compete clause regulations applicable to NPs in their state.
2. Examine the scope of practice laws for NPs in their state, identifying how these laws influence the terms of an employment contract.
3. Interpret the key provisions of the NPA relevant to their practice.

The NPA establishes the legal scope of practice for NPs and varies from state to state. While all states have an NPA, the specific regulations, including prescriptive authority, independent practice, and supervisory requirements, can differ significantly.

Instructions: Complete the following steps:

1. **Identify legal counsel**: Research and list at least three legal practices in your area or nationally that offer employment contract review services for NPs. Include the typical fee structure for these services and note whether additional fees are charged for negotiating contract terms.
2. **Non-compete restrictions**: Investigate the law in your state related to non-compete clauses for health care providers. Summarize the limitations and conditions under which non-compete agreements are enforceable.

3. **Scope of practice laws**: Review the scope of practice laws for NPs in your state. Summarize the key components, such as prescriptive authority, requirements for collaborative agreements, and limitations on practice.

4. **NPA review**: Download and read the NPA for your state. Identify and discuss three key duties or conditions from the NPA that you would address during employment contract negotiations. Explain why these provisions are important for protecting your practice and professional license.

Rubric:

Criteria	Excellent (4)	Good (3)	Satisfactory (2)	Needs Improvement (1)	Score
Legal Counsel Identification	Thoroughly identifies 3 or more practices with detailed fee structures and negotiation fees.	Identifies 2 practices with general fee details.	Identifies 1 practice with limited fee details.	Does not identify any practices or fee details are missing.	/4

(continued)

(continued)

Criteria	Excellent (4)	Good (3)	Satisfactory (2)	Needs Improvement (1)	Score
Non-Compete Restrictions	Provides a comprehensive analysis of state laws with clear implications for NPs.	Provides a good summary of state laws.	Provides a basic summary with some inaccuracies.	Provides an incomplete or inaccurate summary.	/4
Scope of Practice Laws	Offers a detailed summary of state laws with implications for practice.	Offers a general overview of state laws.	Provides a minimal overview, lacking key details.	Little to no information about state laws.	/4

NPA Review and Contract Conditions	Identifies and justifies 3 relevant duties from NPA with a clear rationale for negotiation.	Identifies 2 relevant duties with general rationale.	Identifies 1 duty with limited justification.	Does not identify relevant duties or lacks justification. /4
Organization and Clarity	Clear, well-organized, and free of grammatical errors.	Mostly clear with minor errors.	Somewhat clear but with noticeable errors.	Lacks clarity and has multiple errors. /4
Total Score				/20

Assignment #2: Negotiation for Novice NPs

Goal: To develop and practice contract negotiation skills specific to NP employment agreements.

Objectives:

1. **Analyze** the components of a standard NP employment contract and identify negotiable and non-negotiable terms.
2. **Develop** a negotiation strategy by creating a list of priorities and formulating counterarguments for the employer's potential responses.
3. **Demonstrate** effective negotiation techniques by role-playing a mock negotiation session, advocating for personal interests while considering the employer's constraints.

Instructions:

Pair up with a fellow NP student. Decide who will play the role of the NP candidate and who will act as the employer.

Create a fictional job offer scenario. Include details such as:

- **Salary**: Base pay, potential bonuses, or raises.
- **Benefits**: Health insurance, PTO.
- **Termination clause**: Conditions under which the contract can be terminated by either party.
- **CME**: Allowances or days off for professional development.

Scenario:

Each student should develop a written negotiation plan, outlining their primary objectives, potential employer responses, and prepared counterarguments. Consider the following when preparing the strategy:

- What are your non-negotiables (e.g., minimum salary)?
- What areas are you willing to compromise on (e.g., specific benefits)?
- What arguments or evidence can you present to support your requests?

Mock Negotiation:

During the mock negotiation session, both students should remain in their assigned roles throughout the exercise. The NP candidate should clearly articulate their terms, advocating for their personal interests and priorities. Meanwhile, the employer should take into account their own constraints, such as budget limitations and organizational priorities, and respond accordingly to the NP candidate's proposals.

Debrief and Reflection:

After the negotiation, engage in a discussion with your partner to reflect on the experience. Consider what strategies were effective in advocating for your

(continued)

(continued)

interests, the challenges you faced during the negotiation, and how you addressed them. Additionally, discuss how this exercise mirrored real-world contract negotiations and what insights can be applied to future scenarios.

Write a brief reflection (200 words approx.) on what you learned from this experience and how you would approach future negotiations differently.

Rubric

Criteria	Exemplary (5 pts)	Proficient (4 pts)	Basic (3 pts)	Needs Improvement (2 pts)	Unsatisfactory (1 pt)
Scenario Development	Comprehensive scenario with detailed terms and context.	Detailed scenario with most key terms included.	Basic scenario with some key terms but lacks detail.	Limited scenario, missing key components.	Minimal or no scenario details provided.
Negotiation Strategy	Thorough strategy with clear objectives and counterarguments.	Clear strategy with most objectives and counterarguments.	Strategy outlined, but missing some objectives or arguments.	Limited strategy with few objectives and arguments.	No clear strategy or objectives presented.

Criteria					
Mock Negotiation Performance	Demonstrates strong advocacy and adaptability in negotiation.	Advocates effectively, showing some adaptability.	Basic advocacy, limited adaptability.	Minimal advocacy, struggles with adaptability.	No advocacy or engagement in the negotiation.
Reflection and Debrief	In-depth reflection with clear learning points and future plans.	Clear reflection with some learning points and future plans.	Basic reflection, limited learning points or future plans.	Minimal reflection, lacks learning points or future plans.	No reflection or insights presented.
Professionalism and Role-Playing	Consistently professional, stays in character throughout.	Mostly professional, occasionally breaks character.	Basic professionalism, frequent breaks in character.	Limited professionalism, often out of character.	No professionalism, no role-play engagement.

Total: 25 points

4.2   Conclusion

Understanding the intricacies of an NP job contract is important for ensuring a rewarding and sustainable career. By familiarizing oneself with key contract terms, reviewing the offer, and negotiating effectively, the NP can secure a position that aligns with one's professional goals and personal needs. It is recommended one seek professional advice when needed. Additional factors to consider include compensation for on-call duties and hospital rounds, as these should be proportionate to what other providers in the practice receive. For salaried positions, benefits such as health insurance, vacation time, sick leave, travel allowance, continuing education support, malpractice insurance, and professional memberships should be negotiated. It's also essential to ensure that the job allows you to practice fully within your scope, without unnecessary restrictions or expectations to perform beyond your legal scope of practice.

References

1. Brown, M. and Dolan, M. (2016). Employment contracts for nurse practitioners: understanding the essentials. *JNP* 41 (3): 14–19.
2. Buppert, C. (2023). *The Nurse Practitioner's Business Practice and Legal Guide*, 8the. Jones & Bartlett Learning.
3. Dolan, C.M. (2017). Understanding employment contracts: What to know before you sign. *Nurse Pract.* 42 (11): 44–49. https://doi.org/10.1097/01.NPR.0000521996.45934.ba. PMID: 29040178.
4. American Association of Nurse Practitioners (2024). Employment negotiations: Don't forget these things when considering a position. https://www.aanp.org/practice/practice-management/employment-negotiations (accessed 7 October 2024).

5. Scott, C., Sackmaster, S., Schembre, D. et al. Best Practice recommendation: advanced proactice providers contract terms and negotiations. *IIE* 2 (3): 395–398, ISSN: 2949-7086, https://doi.org/10.1016/j.igie.2023.07.004. Accessed 10 October 2024.

6. Ryan, LLC v. Federal Trade Commission. (2024). No. 3:24-cv-00986 (N.D. Tex. Aug. 20, 2024). U.S. Chamber Reply Brief - Ryan v. FTC, N.D. Tex. https://www.uschamber.com/assets/documents/U.S.-Chamber-Reply-Brief-Ryan-v.-FTC-N.D.-Tex.pdf (accessed 7 October 2024).

7. Marshall, J., Ashwath, M., Jefferies, J. et al. (2023). Restrictive covenants and noncompete clauses for physicians. *JACC Adv.* 2 (7): 100547. https://doi.org/10.1016/j.jacadv.2023.100547.

8. Tyler, L. A., and Weiss, L. A. (2020). Salary, benefits packages, and negotiation skills for nurse practitioners [Doctor of Nursing Practice Scholarly Project, Pittsburg State University]. Pittsburg State University Digital Commons. https://digitalcommons.pittstate.edu/dnp/43 (accessed 12, October, 2024).

9. American Association of Nurse Practitioners (2022). Employment contracts for nurse practitioners: What to consider. https://www.aanp.org (accessed 7 October 2024).

Chapter 5

Launching Into Practice: The Inaugural Year

Sara L. Gleasman-DeSimone PhD, ANP-C

Le Moyne College, Graduate Nursing Department, Syracuse, NY, USA

NP Transition to Practice Reflection
Katherine Halstead, DNP, FNP-C
Le Moyne College, Graduate Nursing Department, Syracuse, NY, USA

Nurse Practitioner: Transition Guide, First Edition. Sara L. Gleasman-DeSimone.
© 2025 John Wiley & Sons, Inc. Published 2025 by John Wiley & Sons, Inc.

Chapter Highlights

Transitioning to Practice
Clinical Competence and Benner's Model
Imposter Syndrome and Strategies to Overcome
Onboarding and Credentialing Essentials
Importance of Effective Time Management
Legal and Regulatory Compliance for NPs

5.1   Introduction

What an exciting time this is! The transition from a student to a practicing nurse practitioner (NP) is a significant phase that requires preparation and a deep understanding of both professional and clinical aspects. These are big steps and can be challenging! Successfully adjusting to the role of an NP is essential for several reasons. It ensures that new NPs are equipped to deliver high-quality, patient-centered care. This progression helps build strong professional relationships with colleagues, fostering a supportive work environment. It also allows new NPs to handle challenges like imposter syndrome (IP) and burnout, thereby protecting their well-being. Ultimately, making a smooth transition lays the groundwork for a fulfilling and sustainable career, enabling new NPs to excel in their role! This chapter is designed to guide new NPs through this journey, offering insights into essential topics such as managing imposter syndrome, onboarding and credentialing, legal and regulatory requirements, and effective time management. Let's continue the journey!

Chapter Objectives and Mapping to 2021 AACN Essentials

1. Analyze the impact of imposter syndrome on new NPs and develop strategies to build confidence and professional identity. Domain 2: Person-Centered Care. Domain 9: Professionalism.
2. Identify some key steps involved in the onboarding and credentialing process. Domain 7: Systems-Based Practice Domain 10: Personal, Professional, and Leadership Development.
3. Describe legal and regulatory constraints that impact NP practice. Domain 7: Systems-Based Practice. Domain 9: Professionalism.
4. Evaluate various strategies for adhering to ethical standards and navigating ethical dilemmas in clinical practice. Domain 2: Person-Centered Care. Domain 9: Professionalism.
5. Explain and apply principles from time management theories to NP practice. Domain 5: Quality and Safety. Domain 10: Personal, Professional, and Leadership Development.

5.2   Understanding the Transition Process

"Change is the end result of all true learning."

—Leo Buscaglia

As a new NP steps into practice, every challenge faced marks a stride toward continuous improvement. The evolution of an NP from the registered nurse (RN) role to a provider is a particularity challenging time. The transition involves a shift from being an RN to managing patients, including diagnosing and treating, prescribing medications, and focusing on health promotion and disease prevention. Foundational nursing values of caring, empathy, and advocacy are preserved and offer patients a unique perspective as an NP. Challenges in the first year of practice involve balancing these new roles with the psychological adjustments necessary to perform effectively.

5.3   NP Transition to Practice Reflection

By Katherine Halstead DNP, FNP-C

I am currently an NP and serve as New York State's Health and Wellness Manager at National Grid. Before this, I worked as an NP at a small family practice where I cared for patients ranging from newborns to geriatric individuals. My healthcare experience includes nursing roles in medical/surgical, spinal cord injuries, cardiology, and volunteer Emergency Medical Technician (EMT).

My inspiration to pursue a career in the medical field stems from my sister, Bridget. Bridget underwent six open-heart surgeries. The exceptional care provided by the doctors and nurses to my family motivated me to do the same for others. Building strong rapport with families and patients is incredibly important to me. I live by the principle, "Treat every patient as if they are your family." I often ask myself, "How would I want my mom, dad, grandma, or siblings to be treated?" I believe this mindset is crucial in fostering a positive provider–patient relationship.

When I embarked on my career journey—first as a new RN and later as a new NP—I anticipated a steep learning curve. I consistently asked questions and utilized available resources. This approach significantly boosted my confidence during the first few months of each new role. Reaching out to other providers in various specialties also reassured me that I was on the right track with patient care and helped facilitate collaboration. My first year as an NP was the most challenging as I adapted to the workflow in a family practice setting, which differed significantly from the hospital environment I had been accustomed to for six years.

My advice to graduating NPs is to be kind to yourself. The beginning will be a learning curve, but you will get there. Know your limits and have open conversations with your managers and fellow providers about how many patients you feel comfortable managing. Keep learning—seek out every available opportunity for growth, even if it seems intimidating. Remember that you are making a difference in someone's life, and be proud of all that you have accomplished.

5.4   Clinical Competence

Clinical competence is effectively applying medical knowledge and skills in real-world healthcare settings [1]. While academic training in an NP program establishes a foundational knowledge base, the first year in clinical practice continues to refine these skills. Benner's model of skill acquisition fits nicely in this learning curve with developing clinical competence. Benner's model highlights that real-world experiences are vital for transforming theoretical knowledge into practical expertise [1].

5.4.1 Benner's Model

Patricia Benner's novice to expert model provides a framework for understanding nursing expertise progression through various stages of experience. This model has five levels of nursing experience: novice, advanced beginner, competent, proficient, and expert. Each level represents a different stage in the development of knowledge and decision-making skills [1]. This model is influential because it emphasizes the importance of experiential learning and provides a pathway for professional development by accumulating clinical knowledge via practical experience. It supports the notion that professional growth is possible by moving through these stages of development.

5.4.1.1 Progression

Novices are beginners with no practical experience and strictly follow detailed rules based on textbook learning [1]. Advanced beginners gain a working level of competence by applying their growing experiential knowledge to real situations, though they still can rely heavily on guidelines. The competent stage, typically achieved after two to three years in a specific clinical role, sees nurses developing strong organizational and planning abilities. They view their actions within the framework of long-term goals and plans, becoming more aware of these goals and working more efficiently toward them. They begin to handle the complexities and unpredictability of clinical situations with greater ease. Proficient nurses perceive and understand situations holistically and make decisions that reflect the understanding of what is needed for long-term outcomes. This draws from their wealth of experience. Experts operate at an advanced level characterized by intuitive and highly adaptive responses to complex clinical situations. At this point, there is less requirement of rules and analytical tools, relying instead on a profound, instinctual understanding of the clinical environment.

5.4.1.2   NP Transitioning Through Benner's Framework

Patricia Benner's framework from novice to expert provides a valuable structure for understanding the development of clinical competence in NPs [1]. NPs in the novice stage can tend to follow protocols and procedures strictly due to their limited experience. For example, the new NP managing high blood pressure may follow the standard guidelines, prescribing first-line medications and looking at comorbidities like kidney disease. In the advanced beginner stage, NPs start to recognize patterns and early signs of treatment resistance or side effects, which allows them to recognize other factors and make minor adjustments. During this time, there is still a reliance on guidelines with decision-making but the new NP still seeks guidance from seasoned providers [1].

At the competent level, typically achieved after a few years in practice, NPs can more efficiently manage their workload and are better at prioritizing patient visits with increased autonomy. They are equipped to coordinate care across different specialties and anticipate potential complications [1]. For instance, a more competent NP might develop a comprehensive care plan for a patient with multiple chronic conditions, integrating insights from various specialties they collaborate with. Proficient NPs develop a deeper holistic understanding of disease progression which enables them to be more intuitive and to adjust treatment plans with ease.

Finally, as experts, NPs demonstrate a high degree of clinical fluency, handling emergencies with precision.

Their extensive experience and knowledge provide tailored patient care, often identifying and addressing issues before they become critical. For example, an expert NP might intervene early in a deteriorating patient's condition, using their extensive experience to adjust treatment plans effectively while still following clinical guidelines.

5.4.2   The Role of Experiential Learning and Reflection

Kolb's (1984) experiential learning cycle describes how individuals learn through a continuous process involving four key stages [2]. These stages begin with concrete experience, where one engages directly in a specific activity or situation. This is followed by reflective observation, where individuals reflect on the experience to understand what happened and why. Next, abstract conceptualization involves developing theories or principles based on those reflections. Finally, in active experimentation, individuals apply these new insights to new situations to refine. This cycle promotes ongoing learning.

Kolb's experiential learning cycle and Benner's stages can work well together. Both provide an approach to support continuous learning and growth. Clinical competence involves this process and sets the framework for growth in practice. The new NP can continue to reflect on their stages and how they handled the day-to-day situations. This creates meaning and understanding of this normal process.

5.4.2.1   NP Application

As NPs progress through Benner's stages, each phase can be enriched by Kolb's cycle. For instance, a novice NP might handle a complex case of managing a patient with multiple chronic conditions, such as diabetes and hypertension.

The experience of coordinating care for this patient includes conducting a physical assessment, implementing a treatment, and scheduling follow-ups. Reflection involves the NP analyzing how they approached care, evaluating what strategies were practical, and identifying areas for improvement. In the abstract conceptualization stage, the NP takes these reflections to refine and continue to manage these conditions more effectively. Active experimentation involves applying this new approach in future cases, such as tailoring interventions based on insights gained from previous experiences and building with each patient. The outcome is managing complex cases more effectively. This can take time, but the process is supported along the way.

Benner's model emphasizes the value of learning from real-world clinical experiences, especially those that push practitioners beyond their comfort zones. Kolb's cycle helps NPs analyze these experiences, extract meaningful insights, and apply them to future patients and practice. Suggested reflective practices such as journaling or debriefing with mentors would help the NP validate and reflect for continuous improvement.

5.4.3 Embracing Challenges

In addition to reflection, embracing the fact that challenges are not going away will assist in a proactive approach to clinical competence. Setbacks are a reality, and NPs should view them as opportunities for growth and not failures. This mindset can assist in building resilience as healthcare is uncertain and unpredictable at times. The journey is multifaceted. It's not just overcoming each setback but learning from challenges along the way, so keep up the great work!

5.4.3.1 Bridging Clinical Competence and Psychological Challenges

As NPs strive to develop clinical competence and navigate the challenges of their first year, they often encounter psychological challenges that can undermine their confidence. One such challenge is imposter syndrome (IP), a psychological pattern where individuals doubt their accomplishments and are afraid of being exposed as a fraud [3]. Despite their success in their academic program and hard-earned skills, those experiencing imposter syndrome feel inadequate and believe their achievements are due to luck rather than abilities. This phenomenon is widespread in high-achieving professions, especially transitioning from education to real-world practice settings. Addressing imposter syndrome is a must for NPs to fully utilize their clinical skills and develop the self-assurance needed to thrive in their roles.

5.5   Imposter Syndrome

The concept of imposter syndrome, originally termed the "imposter phenomenon," was first introduced by psychologists Dr. Pauline R. Clance and Dr. Suzanne A. Imes in 1978 [3]. Clance and Imes explored the feelings of self-doubt and feeling like a fraud among high-achieving women. Despite success, these women thought they weren't as competent as others perceived. They felt like imposters with a fear of failure. Some of these feelings were linked to their early family experiences or expectations of society. This study led to more research on imposter syndrome across many other professions.

5.5.1   Prevalence and Impact

Imposter syndrome is a significant issue affecting many professionals, including those in the medical field. For example, up to 60% of medical students experience imposter syndrome [4]. Far from being a short phase, imposter syndrome has been known to lead to burnout and overall poor mental health. A high-pressure culture in the medical field exacerbates these feelings, particularly among women and minority groups who have been known to face additional societal and structural barriers [5, 6]. The prevalence of imposter syndrome is well-documented across various professions and can impact mental health, job satisfaction, and self-efficacy [7, 8].

There is a connection between the imposter phenomenon and maladaptive perfectionism that can lead to psychological distress [9]. Maladaptive perfectionism strives to be flawless but sets unrealistic standards and can tend to be overly critical of themselves. Those suffering from imposter syndrome frequently display unhealthy perfectionist behaviors while trying to always be in control. These tendencies can intensify feelings of being an imposter and adversely affect overall mental health. There is a need to address imposter syndrome and perfectionism in different settings to help people with coping mechanisms to reduce the mental health impacts. One way is to review the contributing factors.

5.5.2   Contributing Factors

Imposter syndrome in medical professionals is often triggered by several factors, which can exacerbate feelings of self-doubt and inadequacy. For example, the nature of medical training and practice can foster a culture where mistakes can be highly scrutinized, leading to heightened self-doubt among those learning professionals. These high expectations create an environment where medical practitioners feel immense pressure to perform without flaw. Additionally, women and minority medical professionals can frequently encounter bias and microaggressions from others, which reinforce feelings of inadequacy and the belief that their successes are due to luck and not skill [10]. These experiences of gender and racial bias further contribute to imposter syndrome. Significant transitions, such as moving from the academic setting to clinical or residency, often intensify feelings of being an imposter as individuals adjust to new responsibilities and environments. These transitions demand rapid adaptation to new roles and expectations, making it challenging for medical professionals to feel confident in their abilities.

5.5.3   Application to New Nurse Practitioners

New NPs are susceptible to imposter syndrome, particularly as they transition from education to clinical practice. They may doubt their clinical decisions and fear mistakes despite their training and knowledge. This can lead to an overreliance on colleagues for confirmation and hinder their confidence in making independent decisions. Additionally, new NPs might attribute positive patient outcomes to other factors such as team support or luck rather than skills. This perpetuates feelings of fraudulence and diminishing self-esteem [11]. As a result, they might shy away from complex cases or defer to more experienced practitioners, which can limit their professional growth [7].

To help mitigate these effects, it's helpful for healthcare organizations to implement supportive onboarding programs with mentorship and continuous learning opportunities. These programs should include a strong emphasis on mental health and well-being. By addressing imposter syndrome proactively, organizations can help new NPs build confidence, reduce the risk of burnout, and ensure a more effective and satisfying professional journey [12].

5.5.4   Overcoming Imposter Syndrome

To help overcome imposter syndrome, several proactive strategies can be effective. For example, mentorship programs, where new NPs are paired with experienced mentors who provide guidance, feedback, and reassurance, can be helpful. Mentors can share their own experiences with imposter syndrome, normalizing these feelings and offering coping strategies [13]. Professional development workshops that focus on building confidence, resilience, and self-awareness can equip NPs with tools to recognize and combat imposter syndrome. Techniques such as cognitive-behavioral strategies and mindfulness can also be helpful [14]. Creating a supportive work environment that values questions and learning can reduce the fear of being judged, helping new NPs feel more comfortable in their roles and validating their competencies [15]. NPs can address specific weaknesses by reading about diseases or conditions to close knowledge gaps head-on. It's also important for NPs to expect peaks and valleys in their learning journey and use their foundational knowledge to build on.

5.5.4.1   Organizational Support/Onboarding Programs

Erickson et al. (2021) explored the importance of establishing robust organizational support systems to facilitate the transition of NPs into practice [16]. Their research underscores the necessity of structured transition programs that encompass mentorship, phased integration of clinical duties, and clear communication of expectations. By incorporating these elements, healthcare organizations can reduce turnover rates, increase job satisfaction, and ensure high-quality patient care. Such programs are crucial for addressing new NPs' clinical and emotional needs, fostering a supportive environment that promotes professional growth and smooths the transition into practice [16].

Ortiz Pate et al. (2022) identified successful strategies for onboarding NPs and PAs in primary care settings, emphasizing mentorship, continuous education, and tailored patient scheduling [17]. Consistent education and skills training with onboarding ensure that NPs are well-prepared to handle clinical responsibilities in practice as there is a learning curve. Mentorship programs provide guidance and support, helping new practitioners build their professional identities and navigate the complexities of their roles. Orienting new NPs to the organizational culture and team structure helps them integrate smoothly into the workplace.

Tailoring patient scheduling to allow for a gradual increase in responsibilities can also help new NPs adjust to their roles more effectively. For example, scheduling two patients an hour for a month, increasing as the NP gets used to the practice, Electronic Medical Record (EMR), and flow. This will ensure a smoother transition and not overwhelm the provider. These measures not only improve job satisfaction and retention rates but contribute to the overall quality of healthcare delivery [16, 17].

5.5.4.2 Workshop Strategies

Haney et al. (2018) conducted a workshop to address the impact of imposter syndrome on clinical nurse specialists [18]. The workshop's primary objective was to create a forum for discussing the various impacts of imposter syndrome on professional practice and personal well-being among healthcare providers. The workshop involved several key activities designed to help participants better understand imposter syndrome. It began with an overview of imposter syndrome, including its definition, common symptoms, and its psychological and professional implications for those affected. Participants were encouraged to share their experiences with imposter syndrome, creating a supportive environment for open discussion. This sharing of personal stories helped to normalize the experience of imposter syndrome and reduce any stigma associated with it.

Next, the workshop focused on the specific impacts, such as increased anxiety, decreased job satisfaction, and impaired performance. It introduced several strategies including cognitive-behavioral techniques to challenge these negative thought patterns, mentorship reinforcement, and the development of a supportive professional network. Participants engaged in role-playing exercises to practice these strategies and received feedback from peers and facilitators.

The workshop concluded with a reflection session during which participants discussed their key takeaways and how they planned to implement the strategies in their professional lives [18]. Overall, the workshop provided valuable insights and practical tools to understand and mitigate the effects of imposter syndrome, fostering a more supportive and empowering professional environment.

5.5.4.3 Application to NP's

The workshop approach can effectively help NPs to help manage and overcome imposter syndrome [18]. This can be simulated in the academic environment before graduation to prepare for this or in a practice setting to support the new providers. By integrating these workshops into professional development programs, healthcare institutions can enhance the mental well-being of NPs, reduce feelings of inadequacy, and promote a culture of resilience and self-efficacy among new practitioners.

5.5.4.4 Mentorship and Guidance

Establishing mentorship programs that pair new NPs with experienced colleagues can provide essential guidance, share valuable experiences, and offer reassurance [19]. NPs should be encouraged to seek individual mentors within their workplace or professional networks for personalized support in navigating their roles. Mentors are usually accessible in one's workplace with more experience that one can go to with questions. Additionally, facilitating peer support groups where NPs can engage in open discussions, share experiences, and provide mutual support can alleviate feelings of isolation and validate shared challenges [19]. Promoting attendance at conferences and workshops tailored to NP roles is helpful for staying updated and networking. Be grateful for the mentor's time and remember not to ask questions that one can easily look up!

5.6 Conclusion

Addressing imposter syndrome among new NPs requires a comprehensive and multifaceted approach incorporating personal strategies and institutional support. By implementing structured onboarding programs, fostering a supportive culture, and providing continuous professional development opportunities, healthcare organizations can help new NPs navigate their transition more effectively. Workshops and mentorship programs should be specifically designed to address the challenges of imposter syndrome. This can empower NPs to build confidence, reduce feelings of inadequacy, and enhance their professional growth. Ultimately, these efforts will lead to improved job satisfaction, better mental health, and higher quality of patient care, benefiting both practitioners and the healthcare system.

Assignment #1   Imposter Syndrome

Goal: To help students/new NPs understand imposter syndrome and apply strategies to help overcome this issue.

Objectives:

1. Identify the characteristics and manifestations of imposter syndrome.
2. Analyze a scenario where imposter syndrome might affect clinical decision-making and professional growth.
3. Develop strategies to overcome imposter syndrome.

Assignment Instructions:

Read the scenario on imposter syndrome thoroughly. Reflect on any personal experiences or observations

(continued)

(continued)

related to imposter syndrome, whether in clinical rotations, or other professional settings.

Scenario Analysis: Discuss how imposter syndrome is evident in the scenario and its potential impact on the individual's performance and well-being.

Scenario:

Brian, a new NP, has recently started working in a busy urban clinic. He graduated with top honors and has completed over 1,000 hours in clinical. One morning, Brian sees his first patient presenting with symptoms of a respiratory infection, cough with green sputum, fever, and shortness of breath. Despite his assessment and feeling confident in his clinical skills, he second-guesses the diagnosis. He decides to consult his collaborating physician for confirmation. This pattern of seeking validation continues with almost every patient. Brian feels anxious about making independent decisions and fears he might make a mistake, despite having the required knowledge and training. Over time, this undermines his confidence and slows the decision-making process. He opted to refer the next patient to a more experienced colleague instead of handling it himself. This avoidance of complex cases becomes a pattern in the coming days.

Discussion Questions:

1. How does Brian's behavior exemplify imposter syndrome? Give two examples.
2. What impact might this constant seeking of validation or avoiding challenging cases have on his professional growth and patient care?

Assignment Rubric:

Criteria	Excellent (4)	Good (3)	Fair (2)	Poor (1)	Points
Scenario Analysis	Thorough and insightful analysis of the scenario.	Clear analysis with minor gaps in insight.	Basic analysis with several gaps in understanding.	Minimal analysis, lacking depth and insight.	/4
Reflection and Insight	Demonstrates deep reflection and personal insight.	Demonstrates reflection with some personal insight.	Demonstrates basic reflection with limited personal insight.	Lacks reflection and personal insight.	/4

Total Points: /8

Assignment #2:   Reflection

Goal: To develop self-awareness and improve clinical practice through reflection, enhancing the professional growth and competence of the new NP role.

Objectives:

1. Describe daily clinical experiences to identify positive accomplishments and areas needing improvement.
2. Evaluate personal strengths and gaps in knowledge or skills, determining their impact on clinical practice.
3. Create an action plan for continuous professional development based on reflections.

   Instructions: As a new NP in clinical practice, it's essential to engage in regular self-reflection to develop one's skills and address areas of uncertainty. This reflection log is a tool to help to think about daily experiences and identify strategies for professional growth. This can be done as an NP student in clinical training or a new NP in practice.

   Daily Completion: Fill out the reflection log at the end of each day for 2–5 days. Engage in honest and detailed reflections to gain the most benefit. Review logs to identify patterns of strengths and areas needing improvement. Use the reflections to create actionable steps for continuous learning and professional development. It is recommended to share reflections with a mentor or peer to gain additional insights and support.

Reflection Log with Examples

Reflection Steps and Examples	NP Reflection
1. Positive Accomplishments—Describe a situation where you felt you made a positive impact on a patient today. Any specific actions you took that led to this?	Example: "Today, I successfully diagnosed and treated a patient with Chronic Obstructive Pulmonary Disease (COPD) exacerbation. My thorough assessment and confident decision-making with a solid plan made me feel competent."
2. Personal Strengths—What skills or qualities did you demonstrate today you are proud of? How did these strengths contribute to your effectiveness as an NP?	Example: "I used my communication skills to explain a complex treatment plan for diabetes to my patient. I made sure they understood, and it was a good visit."

(continued)

(continued)

Reflection Steps and Examples	NP Reflection
3. Identifying Gaps—Reflect on a moment where you felt unsure or doubted your abilities. What was the situation and what do you think contributed to your uncertainty?	Example: "I felt unsure when interpreting labs/liver enzymes. What do I do? I was anxious. I sought validation from another provider, which made me feel incompetent. I need to read on liver enzymes more."
4. Learning Opportunities— What new knowledge or skills did you gain today? How will you apply this new knowledge in the future?	Example: "I learned about a new diagnostic tool for respiratory infections. I plan to incorporate this tool into my assessments to improve accuracy."
5. Seeking Guidance— Was there a moment today when you sought help, asked a question? How did this moment help you and what did you learn from it?	Example: "I consulted with my collaborating physician about a COPD exacerbation. Their guidance helped me understand the diagnosis process better and gave me confidence for future COPD exacerbations."

Reflection Steps and Examples	NP Reflection
6. Action Plan for Improvement— Identify one specific area where you want to improve based on these experiences. List at least one actionable step to address this area and time frame for implementation.	Example: "I need to improve my confidence in interpreting lab results (liver enzymes). Plan: (1) Review lab interpretation guidelines weekly. (2) Attend a conference on advanced diagnostics. (3) Practice with case studies."

Clinical Reflection Log for New Nurse Practitioners

Reflection Steps	NP Reflection
Positive Accomplishments— Describe a situation where you felt you made a positive impact on a patient today. Any specific actions you took that led to this?	
Personal Strengths—What skills or qualities did you demonstrate today you are proud of? How did these strengths contribute to your effectiveness as an NP	

(continued)

(continued)

Reflection Steps	NP Reflection
Identifying Gaps—Reflect on a moment where you felt unsure or doubted your abilities. What was the situation and what do you think contributed to your uncertainty?	
Learning Opportunities—What new knowledge or skills did you gain today? How will you apply this new knowledge in the future?	
Seeking Guidance—Was there a moment today when you sought help, asked a question? How did this moment help you and what did you learn from it?	
Action Plan for Improvement—Identify one specific rea where you want to improve based on these experiences. List at least one actionable step to address this area and time frame for implementation.	

5.7   Onboarding and Credentialing

5.7.1   Introduction

The initial steps of onboarding and credentialing are essential for both the organization and the NP to make a smooth transition and integration into the new role. For the organization, the onboarding process involves completing human resource documentation, enrollment of benefits, verifying the NP's credentials, and providing an orientation that covers the organization's policies, procedures, and culture. Likely, the NP already met the team during the interview process, toured the facility, and was made aware of the company's mission and values. Additionally, the organization must ensure the NP's proficiency with their electronic health record (EHR) system, specific clinical protocols, and workflows including the daily schedule, and hopefully assign a mentor to help through the process. Building relationships with colleagues, identifying areas for additional training, and being open to feedback are vital. The next section will review the comprehensive steps of onboarding and credentialing to establishing readiness to practice in the new role.

5.7.2   Credentialing Process

Credentialing involves verifying the qualifications, professional background, and competencies of healthcare providers to ensure they meet the standards required to practice in a healthcare organization [20]. The process aims to confirm that healthcare providers have the necessary education, licensure, and certifications to practice. Additionally, it ensures compliance with state and federal regulations and accreditation standards while establishing a provider's professional history, including any malpractice claims, disciplinary actions, or gaps in employment. The overall outcome of credentialing is the confirmation that the healthcare provider is qualified to practice within the healthcare organization and with a specific patient population.

Credentialing is an essential process overseen by a medical staff office or a credentialing department within an organization. This department meticulously verifies the healthcare providers' qualifications, licenses, certifications, and professional experiences to ensure they meet the required standards for providing care within the facility [21].

5.7.2.1 Practice Settings

NPs are credentialed in various healthcare settings, highlighting their versatile roles in the medical field. These environments include hospitals, outpatient clinics, private practices, urgent care centers, long-term care facilities, home healthcare, community health centers, and telehealth services. Credentialing in these diverse settings ensures that NPs can deliver comprehensive care, manage various patient needs, and maintain professional standards across different areas of healthcare.

5.7.2.2 Steps in Credentialing

1. Verify education and certification
2. Obtain licensure verification/federal/state guidelines
3. Privileging (if hospital based)
4. Competence evaluation
5. Obtain DEA and NPI numbers
6. Insurance credentialing

7. Complete background checks
8. Peer and Professional References

5.7.2.3   Ensuring Excellence and Safety

Credentialing is crucial for several reasons, primarily ensuring patient safety by verifying that nurse practitioners possess the necessary knowledge, skills, and experience to provide safe and effective care. This rigorous process helps maintain high-quality care standards by confirming that NPs have undergone extensive training and hold current certifications [20, 21]. Credentialing also ensures compliance with state and federal regulations and accreditation standards set by organizations such as The Joint Commission and the National Committee for Quality Assurance, further reinforcing the quality of care provided. These processes facilitate reimbursement from insurance companies such as Medicare and Medicaid by ensuring that NPs meet the necessary legal requirements [22].

Credentialing builds trust and credibility with patients and the public, demonstrating a healthcare provider's and organization's commitment to maintaining high care standards. Professional groups such as the Medical Group Management Association provide resources and guidelines that shape how credentialing is conducted. They collectively uphold care standards, ensuring compliance with regulations to safeguard both patients and healthcare organizations [22].

5.7.2.4   Education and Licensing Verification

Ensuring that new NPs have the education required to practice legally and effectively is essential for meeting all legal and professional standards [20]. Credentialing confirms that NPs have graduated from accredited NP programs and possess current certifications from nationally recognized certifying bodies such as the American Nurses Credentialing Center or the American Academy of Nurse Practitioners Certification Board. These certifications attest that NPs have completed rigorous training and evaluations, demonstrating comprehensive expertise in specialized areas such as acute care, family practice, pediatrics, or other specialties. Second, licensure verification ensures that NPs hold active and unrestricted RN licenses in the state where they intend to practice as NPs. A comprehensive credentialing review involves reviewing this educational background, additional training, or fellowships (if any), licenses, and often includes professional references and background checks [20].

5.7.2.5   Competencies and Background Checks

The credentialing process involves a comprehensive evaluation of competencies to ensure the new NP is equipped to provide safe, effective, and high-quality patient care. This thorough evaluation includes components such as peer reviews, faculty evaluations, and assessments of clinical outcomes [23]. These measures are essential for confirming that NPs possess the clinical skills and knowledge required for their roles and help healthcare organizations ensure care standards are met [24]. In addition to assessing clinical skills, the credentialing process includes background checks to evaluate an NP's professional conduct history. This involves investigating any previous disciplinary actions, malpractice claims, or legal issues that could affect their ability to practice safely [23]. By reviewing these components, healthcare organizations aim to uphold ethical standards, enhance patient safety, and maintain professional integrity.

5.7.2.6   Sample Credentialing Checklist

Item	Complete
Practitioner Name/Title	✓
Application Complete and Signed	
Professional/Peer References Received	✓
Immunizations/Fit Testing if Applicable	
Health Clearance/Attestation	
Education Verification	
Work History	✓
Residence/Address	
Certifications	
License/State	
Fellowships if Applicable	
Other Education	
DEA Confirmed	
Federation of State Medical Boards Queried	
Criminal Background	
Malpractice History (If Claim—Explanation)	
NPI	
Liability Coverage	
Insurance Forms	
Medicare Attestation Signature Page	

Note: This checklist is for illustrative/educational purposes only.

These steps involve defining the specific clinical privileges and responsibilities that align with the NP's qualifications in various healthcare settings, such as hospitals or clinics [24]. These decisions ensure that NPs operate within their scope of practice, comply with regulations, and contribute effectively to patient care.

5.7.2.7 Obtaining a DEA Number

Obtaining a Drug Enforcement Administration (DEA) number is a fundamental step for new NPs to be legally authorized to prescribe controlled substances. This process ensures that NPs comply with federal regulations and maintain the legal authority necessary for their prescribing duties [25]. To begin the process, NPs must visit the Department of Justice website and select the appropriate application form for their profession and state of practice [26]. The application requires the submission of personal information, professional credentials, and details of the NP's practice location. Additionally, the application fee is around eight hundred dollars for three years, and the processing time for receiving a DEA number typically ranges from four to six weeks [25]. In some cases, the NP's employing organization may handle the DEA number application process on their behalf; however, it is often the NP's responsibility to complete the application independently [26]. Once the application is approved, the DEA issues a unique DEA number, which authorizes the NP to prescribe controlled substances within the scope of their practice [25].

5.7.2.8 DEA Training Requirements for Nurse Practitioners

As of June 27, 2023, new regulations require all DEA-registered practitioners, including NPs, to complete a one-time, eight-hour training focused on treating and managing patients with substance use disorders. This requirement, established by the Medication Access and Training Expansion (MATE) Act, seeks to enhance practitioners' abilities to address the opioid crisis and manage substance use disorders effectively [27].

Under the Consolidated Appropriations Act of 2023, enacted on December 29, 2022, the MATE Act mandated that all DEA-registered practitioners complete this training on substance use disorder treatment and management [26]. This requirement applies to initial registrations and renewals. Practitioners must confirm their completion of the training by checking a box on the DEA registration form, with the training being necessary only once throughout their career [26].

The training must include content on FDA-approved medications treating substance use disorders and can be completed through various accredited programs. These educational programs are designed to provide a foundational understanding of substance use disorder prevention, treatment strategies, and the role of medications in managing these conditions. To meet the requirement, NPs have several options for fulfilling the eight-hour training requirement as many accredited organizations offer this. In addition to these accredited options, there are waived trainings that include past relevant education or training and are automatically considered to meet the requirements [27]. This includes practitioners who are board-certified in addiction medicine or psychiatry, and recent graduates from relevant US medical schools who have completed similar training as part of their education [26].

5.7.2.9   NPI Number

A National Provider Identifier (NPI) is a unique identification number issued by the Centers for Medicare & Medicaid Services (CMS) that is essential for all administrative and financial transactions in the healthcare system [28]. As of May 23, 2007, the Health Insurance Portability and

Accountability Act of 1996 mandated that all healthcare providers obtain an NPI number [28]. This regulation was introduced to streamline administrative processes and improve data accuracy across healthcare systems. By standardizing the identification of healthcare providers, the NPI replaces various identification numbers previously used across different health plans, thereby reducing administrative errors and simplifying care coordination [29].

For NPs, the NPI number is indispensable for several vital functions, including issuing prescriptions, billing for services, and processing insurance claims. NPs employed by a hospital can use the hospital's NPI number when prescribing medications for hospital patients. However, for most other practices, NPs must use their personal NPI number to ensure proper documentation and reimbursement [30].

To obtain an NPI number, NPs must complete an application through the National Plan and Provider Enumeration System website, available at https://nppes.cms.hhs.gov/NPPES/Welcome.do. The application requires the NP to provide personal details, information about their practice location, and professional credentials, including a valid state license. Once submitted, the application is generally processed within 10 business days [28].

5.7.3 Privileging

Privileging is granting a healthcare provider the authorization to perform procedures and deliver services within a healthcare organization based on their credentials and demonstrated competence [31]. The purpose of privileging is to ensure that healthcare providers are competent to perform specific clinical tasks and procedures safely and effectively. The steps involved usually include applying for specific clinical privileges, a review of credentials, a competence assessment, and an interview and evaluation by the privileging committee. The outcome of the privileging process is the authorization for the healthcare provider to perform specific procedures and provide specific services. This includes an ongoing monitoring plan with periodic reevaluation and renewal of privileges.

The most common type of privileging is in hospital systems. New NPs secure hospital privileges that include enrolling with insurance companies including Medicare/ Medicaid, offering reimbursable services [31]. This process includes gathering essential documentation, including curriculum vitae (CV), RN and NP licenses, national certification, proof of malpractice insurance, DEA registration, and state-specific controlled substances registration [31]. Most likely the applicant will undergo criminal background checks, drug screenings, and a health history and physical, as mandated by the institution. At times, attending an interview with the hospital's credentialing committee is required to discuss clinical experience and the scope of practice required. The application will undergo review by the committee. This is maintained by keeping licenses and certifications up to date, continuing education requirements, and other procedures as specified. This process ensures that the NP is well-qualified to deliver healthcare procedures and services within the hospital environment.

5.7.3.1 Key Differences Between Credentialing and Privileging

The primary difference between credentialing and privileging lies in the scope and purpose. Credentialing involves verifying the provider's overall qualifications and professional history to ensure they meet the general standards of practice within the organization. In contrast, privileging focuses on granting permission to perform specific clinical tasks and procedures based on qualifications and competence that are verified. Credentialing is the confirmation of the provider's general qualifications, while the outcome of privileging is the specific authorization to perform designated procedures and services. Overall, both processes uphold practice standards, protect patient welfare, and support the professional growth and development of NPs as valuable members of the healthcare team.

5.7.4   Recredentialing

Recredentialing is the fundamental process for NPs to maintain their professional qualifications and continue providing high-quality care in a particular institution. This typically occurs every two to three years, depending on state regulations and the requirements of certifying organizations [32]. The recredentialing process involves several components, including the completion of continuing education relevant to the NP's specialty, documentation of clinical practice hours, and undergoing performance evaluations [33]. Additionally, NPs must provide proof of malpractice insurance, adhere to health screenings, and comply with professional conduct standards to meet expectations [33]. This allows NPs to practice safely and effectively while upholding standards of care.

5.7.4.1   Documentation and Record-Keeping

NPs should maintain documents such as an updated CV detailing their education, certifications, and professional experience [34]. Copies of current RN and NP licenses, national certification documents, and malpractice insurance should be readily accessible and backed up on a computer. Keeping records of completed continuing education activities, performance evaluations, and professional activities such as committee memberships and research projects is also helpful. Some certification bodies will help members organize continuing education credits done through their website. Organizing these documents systematically helps NPs respond promptly to credentialing requests and ensures they can quickly produce their qualifications and maintain ongoing professional development.

5.8   Insurance

NPs typically need to be credentialed with various insurance companies to be eligible to deliver and bill for healthcare services.

5.8.1   Medicare

Medicare, administered by the CMS, offers health insurance primarily to individuals in the United States over 65 and some younger individuals with disabilities [35]. Credentialing with Medicare is an important step for NPs in providing services and receiving reimbursements under this federal health insurance program. To be eligible for Medicare reimbursement, NPs must complete enrollment through the Provider Enrollment, Chain, and Ownership System (PECOS). This process involves submitting the enrollment application with demographics, proof of state licensure, and documentation of malpractice insurance. The application can be accessed through the PECOS website at https://www.cms.gov/Medicare/Provider-Enrollment/ PECOS [35]. The average processing time for Medicare enrollment is approximately 60–90 days, after which the NP receives an NPI number, which is essential for billing Medicare for services rendered [35]. This credentialing process ensures that NPs meet the qualifications to deliver healthcare to Medicare beneficiaries and receive appropriate compensation for their services.

5.8.2   Medicaid

Medicaid is a joint federal and state program in the United States that provides health coverage to eligible low-income individuals and families. The program covers various medical services, including healthcare provider visits, hospital admissions, and long-term care. Medicaid eligibility and benefits can vary from state to state [35].

Unlike Medicare's standardized enrollment process, Medicaid credentialing differs across states, requiring NPs to complete applications specific to their state's Medicaid program. NPs must visit their state's Medicaid office or use the state's Medicaid website to access the application, which requires documentation such as proof of state licensure, malpractice insurance, and background information [35]. The Medicaid enrollment process time can range from 30 to 120 days, depending on the state.

5.8.3   Private Insurance

Credentialing with private insurance companies is a step for NPs to be able to provide services to a broad patient base and receive reimbursement from various insurance plans. To simplify this process, NPs often use the Council for Affordable Quality Healthcare (CAQH) ProView system, which allows them to submit their credentialing information to multiple insurance companies through a single online platform (CAQH) [36].

NPs need to complete a detailed application on the CAQH ProView website when applying for credentialling. Most organizations have the credentialing or billing department do this, and the CAQH ProView system is accessed through the CAQH ProView website at https://proview. caqh.org [36].

This application requires information about the NP's education, licensure, certifications, work history, and malpractice insurance [36]. For example, suppose an NP wants to work with private insurance companies like Blue Cross Blue Shield, UnitedHealthcare, or Aetna. The CAQH ProView system streamlines this process by allowing NPs to enter their information once and share it with multiple insurance companies, making it easier for them to get credentialed with several insurers [36].

For example, UnitedHealthcare is one of the largest health insurance companies in the United States. The process is overseen by the national credentialling committee [37]. This committee reviews applications and makes decisions based on their established criteria. Credentialing is necessary for NPs to treat patients under UnitedHealthcare plans and must be completed before an NP can participate in their network. After the NP receives a notification, they were approved, and they can bill for services with patients currently covered by this insurance [37]. This review process can take anywhere from 90 to 180 days. The process also includes periodic recredentialing to ensure ongoing compliance with standards.

5.9   Billing for Nurse Practitioners

NPs are integral to providing comprehensive healthcare. Effective billing practices ensure that NPs are appropriately compensated for their services. Understanding billing and coding is crucial for navigating insurance requirements and optimizing reimbursement.

5.9.1   Understanding Reimbursement Models and Billing Codes

NPs can be reimbursed through several models, including fee-for-service, capitation, and bundled payments. In a fee-for-service model, reimbursement is based on each service provided, which requires specific numeric coding of procedures and diagnoses. Capitation involves a set fee per patient, per period, regardless of the services rendered, while bundled payments cover all services related to a specific treatment or condition [38].

Billing relies on several coding systems, depending on services, diagnosis, procedures, and place of service. For example, current procedural terminology (CPT) provides codes for describing medical, surgical, and diagnostic services. International Classification of Diseases (ICD) is used for diagnosing a patient condition such as hypertension. The Healthcare Common Procedure Coding System covers additional services and medical supplies [38].

Using the correct codes for diagnoses and treatments is important. For example, when a patient is admitted to the hospital with pneumonia, a specific code like ICD-10 J18.9 is used to document this condition. Similarly, when a patient visits a provider's office, a code like CPT

99213 is used to bill for the office visit. It's important that the diagnosis code (like the ICD-10 code for diabetes) and what was done and documented with the patient that day, match the level of the office visit (like CPT 99213). This ensures that the billing is accurate, and that the healthcare provider receives proper reimbursement. Misalignments between these codes can lead to claim denials, which can delay payment.

To support providers in this process, many healthcare institutions have billing specialists. These professionals assist in selecting the appropriate codes and ensuring that documentation aligns with billing requirements, helping to prevent errors and optimize reimbursement. Proper documentation for each visit or admission is necessary to justify the chosen codes. For more detailed information on medical billing codes, visit www.cms.gov.

5.9.2   Reimbursement and Documentation

Understanding reimbursement policies and maintaining thorough documentation are fundamental for successful billing and compliance. Reimbursement policies can vary significantly by payer; for instance, Medicare reimburses NPs at 85% of the physician fee schedule, while Medicaid rates differ by state [39]. NPs should ensure that patient records reflect all services, diagnoses, and treatments accurately and stay informed about billing regulations and coding updates [38]. Best practices include regularly reviewing billing procedures, using EHR for more precise coding, and consulting billing specialists as needed [38]. Most institutions have billing departments that can help the new NPs with billing codes and periodically review to ensure compliance.

5.10   Conclusion

Credentialing is a comprehensive process that validates the qualifications and legal authority of NPs to provide healthcare services. This involves obtaining necessary licenses, an NPI number, filing for a DEA number, and enrolling in Medicare and Medicaid. Additionally, NPs must complete credentialing with various insurance companies to be recognized as in-network providers for reimbursement. Each step of this process requires careful attention to detail and adherence to regulatory guidelines to ensure that NPs are authorized to practice and can deliver high-quality care. Billing is essential to credentialing as it ensures that NPs are appropriately compensated for their services.

5.11   Time Management

"There is only one success: to be able to spend your life in your own way"

—Christopher Morley

5.11.1   Introduction

I don't have time for all of this!!! Many newer NPs say this after a long day in the clinic or hospital. The first year of an NP's career involves juggling patient encounters, administrative duties, finishing notes, filling prescriptions, triaging sick calls, and delegation. At the same time, maintaining a healthy work-life balance can be difficult. Effective time management is key for new NPs transitioning into their first year of practice. This section will review time management principles and guide how NPs can effectively incorporate these strategies into their practice. This will assist with the

NP's workday management, make it more efficient, and prevent late nights on the computer catching up.

5.11.2   Definition and Problem

Time management is the process of planning and conscious control over the amount of time spent on activities to increase effectiveness and productivity [40]. It involves organizing, scheduling, and prioritizing tasks to make the best use of available time. Effective time management is crucial for productivity and stress reduction, yet many individuals handle tasks as they arise without a structured system. This significantly diminishes their efficiency.

Not having a time management system is a significant error that costs businesses and individuals' valuable time. Research indicates that 82% of people need a proper time management system, leading to only 20% of workers feeling in control of their day [41]. Additionally, the average worker spends over 50% of their workday on low-value tasks that contribute to stress. 39% of US employees attribute their stress to workload [41]. Despite attempting an average of 13 different time management methods, most people still need help finding an effective system. This underscores the importance of time management strategies to enhance satisfaction and productivity. If one dedicates just 10–12 minutes to planning each day, it can save up to two hours, emphasizing the value of time management [41].

5.11.3   Origins of Time Management

Time management has come a long way since it first took shape in the late 19th and early 20th centuries. Frederick Winslow Taylor, in his book *The Principles of Scientific Management*, along with Frank and Lillian Gilbreth, made big changes to how one thinks about productivity by studying how people work, especially in manufacturing. Their approach, known as Taylorism, focused on making work more efficient by standardizing tasks and increasing specialization, which had a huge impact on how organizations were structured. While this approach significantly boosted productivity in manufacturing, it lacked in attention to human interaction and employee satisfaction. This early focus on time management prioritized efficiency and streamlined processes over effectiveness and holistic life balance [42]. This resulted in backlash against this rigid process and led to the human relations movement. It emphasized the importance of worker satisfaction for productivity enhancement. This movement highlighted the need to balance efficiency with employee well-being, promoting a more humane approach to workplace management.

5.11.4   Modern Challenges

In today's time management practices, efficiency and productivity are still the main goals. With all the digital tools available, staying productive is important, but it can sometimes come at the cost of personal interaction and creativity at work [42]. This creates a bit of a tension between pushing for efficiency and maintaining a more human-centered approach. Modern workplaces often focus on getting tasks done quickly and being constantly available, which can limit chances for meaningful conversations and creative thinking.

Despite these challenges, there is a growing interest in approaches that manage internal time and optimize biological clocks to enhance time and life management.

This emerging focus highlights the importance of balancing the historical emphasis on efficiency with overall well-being [42]. By integrating technological advancements with a holistic approach, organizations can create environments that foster productivity while also ensuring individuals' mental and emotional health—a balance crucial for sustainable success in both personal and professional spheres.

5.11.5 Philosophy

Some may still argue that time management begins with a philosophical approach. Philosophy, which is centered on asking questions, plays a crucial role in time management by encouraging individuals to reflect on the most important aspects of their lives [43]. Recognizing time as a finite resource highlights the need to make conscious choices about how it's spent, ensuring that these choices align with personal and professional values. By asking questions like "What tasks are most important?" and "Why am I doing this?" practitioners can clarify their priorities and focus on activities that have the greatest impact. This reflective inquiry also addresses the need for balance, prompting questions such as "How do I balance work and personal life?" which encourages strategies to promote well-being and prevent burnout.

Additionally, questions like "How can I perform this task more efficiently?" drive continuous improvements in workflow and patient care. Ethical considerations are also integral, with inquiries like "Is this the best use of my time for patient outcomes?" guiding decisions in complex clinical situations. This philosophical foundation, rooted in questioning and reflection, enables NPs to have a thoughtful and intentional approach to time management.

5.11.6 *Benefits of Time Management*

Time management has clear benefits, as it is moderately linked to better job performance and overall well-being, while also helping to reduce stress [44]. However, despite these advantages, many people struggle to use time management strategies effectively. There is a need to first understand how effective time management can be in work and life balance.

5.11.6.1 Quality Healthcare

Time management is essential for enhancing clinical efficiency, patient satisfaction, and overall care [44]. It plays a critical role in managing chronic diseases, preventive care, and comprehensive patient evaluations. For NPs, effective time management leads to improved patient outcomes by optimizing schedules and prioritizing tasks. This approach not only enhances patient care but also reduces stress and burnout among NPs. Effective time management can reduce patient wait times, alleviates job-related stress, and ensures that tasks are completed efficiently [45]. Proper time management helps individuals work more efficiently, meet deadlines, produce higher-quality work, and achieve goals faster.

5.11.6.2 Increased Satisfaction and Overall Care

Effective time management also contributes to higher patient satisfaction, closely linked to better patient outcomes. Patients who experienced timely care were more satisfied with their healthcare services [46]. When NPs manage their time well, they can minimize patient wait times while addressing concerns more promptly. Satisfied patients are more likely to adhere to treatment recommendations, attend follow-up appointments, and engage actively in their care, improving health outcomes [47].

Strategic time management also aids NPs in delivering comprehensive and coordinated care, which can also improve patient outcomes. NPs who employ effective time management strategies can better integrate preventive care, coordinate with other healthcare providers, and manage complex patient cases more efficiently. For example, proper time management allows NPs to schedule routine screenings, preventive services, and necessary referrals in a timely manner for early disease detection and comprehensive patient care [48].

5.11.7   Impact of COVID-19 on Time Management for NPs

The COVID-19 pandemic has profoundly affected NPs' time management, introduced new challenges, and reshaped their clinical and personal responsibilities. The pandemic has led to an increased patient load, altered practice environments, and a need for effective time management strategies to maintain work-life balance and continue providing high-quality patient care.

One of the most significant changes has been the increased patient workload and clinical demands. During the pandemic, NPs have faced a surge in patients due to the COVID-19 crisis, which has increased their clinical responsibilities and extended working hours. The need for constant adaptation to changing public health guidelines and the management of COVID-19 cases have contributed to longer shifts and increased stress levels among NPs [49]. This heightened demand has made effective time management essential for NPs to handle their expanded roles without compromising patient care or well-being. The pandemic has also led to significant shifts in practice environments, further complicating time management. Many NPs adjusted to remote telehealth services. This provides new opportunities for patient care but also introduces challenges related to technology and patient engagement [49]. Appointments require different time management skills than traditional in-person visits, as NPs must balance virtual consultations with their in-person responsibilities and manage technical issues [49].

5.11.8 Strategies for Nurse Practitioners

In today's fast-paced healthcare environment, effective time management is essential for NPs to enhance productivity, focus on meaningful tasks, and reduce stress. By adopting specific strategies, NPs can improve their efficiency and job satisfaction while achieving better patient outcomes. Key strategies include focusing on outcomes rather than time, simplifying life with automation, and pre-committing to decisions to reduce fatigue.

Effective time management is crucial for delivering high-quality healthcare, as it ensures that health professionals spend more time with patients, improving care outcomes.

Key factors associated with effective time management included planning skills, staff responsibility, and minimizing time-wasting activities [45]. Identifying and reducing activities that waste time, such as excessive meetings and inefficient communication, can free up more time for patient care [45]. Furthermore, addressing staff shortages and ensuring a supportive work environment are critical for enhancing time management among health professionals [45]. Creating a supportive and well-organized work environment was also emphasized to help health professionals manage their time more effectively. Lastly, research consistently underscores the importance of employee engagement in fostering a productive and innovative work environment. Engaged employees tend to be more committed, motivated, and creative, which can positively impact organizational performance and innovation [50].

5.11.8.1 Automation

Automation can significantly reduce the time spent on repetitive tasks, allowing NPs to focus on more meaningful activities and improve overall patient care. In a healthcare setting, implementing electronic health record (EHR) templates and scheduling software streamlines documentation and administrative tasks, reducing the burden on NPs [51]. For instance, EHR templates can save NPs time by auto-filling routine information, enabling them to focus on patient interactions [52]. Scheduling software like Calendly can streamline appointment booking, reduce administrative overhead, and minimize scheduling conflicts [51]. NPs can enhance their practice efficiency, reduce administrative burdens, and improve overall patient care. Embracing automation not only simplifies daily tasks but also contributes to the well-being and job satisfaction of NPs by allowing them to focus on direct patient care and other critical activities.

5.11.8.2 Electronic Health Records and Block Scheduling

EHR systems with customizable templates allow NPs to quickly document patient encounters by auto-filling standard fields. This system reduces the time spent on documentation and improves accuracy, ensuring that patient records are consistently up-to-date and comprehensive [52]. Additionally, these templates can be tailored to specific clinical workflows and specialties, further enhancing documentation efficiency. By minimizing the time spent on manual data entry, NPs can dedicate more time to direct patient care and other critical tasks, ultimately improving patient outcomes.

The NP can optimize their time by being involved in their scheduling. For example, block scheduling can enable similar patient encounters to focus on specific patient needs. Some electronic medical records can help with this through reminder calls/texts, as well as templates. Incorporating scheduling software to streamline patient appointments is helpful if available. Allocating appropriate time for each patient visit and allowing some reasonable buffer time for unexpected patient needs is useful.

Example

In a busy primary care practice, NP Keisha manages her schedule to enhance efficiency. She schedules new patient appointments for 30 minutes and follow-up visits for 15 minutes. To optimize her time, Keisha uses block scheduling to group similar types of patient encounters. She also allocates a 30-minute slot in the afternoon specifically for handling sick call add-ons. This approach allows her to focus on each type of patient visit more effectively and provides flexibility for unexpected acute cases.

Scheduling software like Calendly automates the scheduling process, allowing patients to book appointments online conveniently. This reduces the administrative burden on NPs and ensures a more organized schedule, minimizing the risk of double bookings and missed appointments. Moreover, automated scheduling tools can send patient reminders, reducing no-show rates and optimizing clinic operations. By streamlining the appointment process, NPs can focus more on patient care and less on administrative tasks.

Platforms like Zapier simplify workflows and decrease manual workload by automating processes such as sending appointment reminders, updating patient records, and managing follow-up communications [53]. Zapier integrates with over 3,000 apps, including popular ones like Gmail, Slack, and Google Sheets, allowing smooth communication between different tools. NPs can create customized workflows, called "Zaps," without coding skills, to automate tasks such as data entry, email notifications, and file backups.

5.11.9   Acceptance with Stoicism

Stoicism, originating in ancient Greece and Roman times, is a philosophy centered on achieving inner tranquility and virtue through rational thinking and disciplined emotion [54]. At its core, Stoicism teaches that happiness is found by accepting what cannot be changed, focusing on personal development, and maintaining a balanced perspective amid life's challenges. This philosophical approach encourages

individuals to cultivate resilience, prioritize what truly matters, and live by principles of reason and virtue rather than
being swayed by external events or emotions.

5.11.9.1   Applying Stoicism to Time Management

Applying Stoic principles to time management involves several strategies. Firstly, accepting what cannot be changed
helps individuals focus their energy on tasks within their
control, enhancing productivity. Prioritizing tasks based on
long-term goals rather than immediate demands effectively
allocates time and resources. Maintaining a balanced perspective fosters clarity and resilience, reducing stress and
enhancing decision-making. Deep focus on one task at a
time, avoiding multitasking distractions, aligns with Stoic
ideals of concentrated effort and excellence. Lastly, adopting a growth mindset, learning from setbacks, and setting
clear, achievable goals keep motivation high and support
continuous improvement [55].

5.11.9.2   Application to Nurse Practitioner Practice

A new NP will encounter a demanding workload and various challenges, making Stoicism a valuable philosophy to
adopt. By accepting the realities of practice that cannot be
changed—such as patient outcomes or specific administrative processes—NPs can better navigate complexities.
Instead of dwelling on these uncontrollable aspects, NPs
should direct their energy toward what they can control,
such as clinical decisions, patient education, and professional growth. Recognizing that the first year will have
peaks and valleys is crucial for developing a sustainable
plan. Additionally, Stoic principles can help prioritize daily
tasks, enhancing efficiency and resilience. Approaching

challenging patient cases or administrative hurdles with a calm and rational mindset enhances decision-making and prevents burnout. This resilience fosters professional growth and enhances the ability to provide quality patient care.

5.11.10   Mere Urgency Effect

Zhu et al. (2018) explored how people often prioritize urgent tasks over important ones, even when the urgency is not objectively warranted [56]. This tendency is termed the "mere urgency effect," illustrating that individuals may choose to complete less important tasks that appear urgent due to an artificial deadline, neglecting tasks with greater significance [56]. Key findings indicate that people are more likely to complete tasks perceived as urgent over those important ones, even when the urgent tasks offer lower rewards. The urgency effect is driven by a focus on time constraints, which can divert the attention from the actual value of the tasks. This mindset can lead to suboptimal decision-making, where essential tasks are procrastinated in favor of completing urgent, less significant ones.

Example

In a psychiatric practice, NP Jamie is faced with an urgent request to call a patient back regarding questions about an appointment. Although this request seems pressing in her lists of tasks, Jamie also needs to complete a detailed assessment for

(continued)

(continued)

a new patient scheduled later that day. By focusing on the urgent issue, Jamie might rush or skip the important assessment, which is essential for planning the new patient's treatment. This shift in focus can result in less effective care for the new patient, showing the importance of balancing urgent tasks with those that have a significant long-term impact.

Recognizing the urgency bias is the first step; being aware of the tendency to prioritize urgent but less important tasks can help make more informed decisions about what truly needs attention. It is essential to focus on the importance of tasks based on their long-term impact on patient care and professional development rather than immediate deadlines. Setting clear priorities using tools like task lists or prioritization grids can help differentiate between urgent and important tasks, ensuring that seemingly urgent but less significant activities do not overshadow critical tasks.

5.11.11   *Work Smarter*

According to Harvard Business Review (2020), time management is more than just using clever tricks [57]. While many resources focus on time management tools, the real challenge is building essential skills that make these tools effective. The key skills are awareness, arrangement, and adaptation. Awareness means recognizing that time is limited and figuring out how much you have. Arrangement is about organizing tasks and goals to be more productive. Adaptation involves adjusting your plans when things don't go as expected or priorities change.

A study with over 1,200 participants tested these time management skills in a simulation and found that awareness, arrangement, and adaptation all matter equally for managing time well. Participants had the most trouble with awareness and adaptation, suggesting these skills are harder to develop and require more focused practice. The study highlights that simply having tools isn't enough; developing self-awareness and key skills is crucial for managing time effectively [57].

Adaptation in time management is all about being flexible when things don't go as planned. It means being able to quickly adjust priorities and tasks when unexpected problems or changes come up. This skill helps one stay focused and keep working efficiently even when interruptions happen. It also involves managing stress and using strategies like time-blocking or productivity tools to help make quick changes. By getting better at adaptation, one can handle challenges more smoothly and be more effective in work and personal life.

5.11.12   Checklists

In "The Checklist Manifesto," Atul Gawande advocates using checklists in medical practice to improve efficiency and patient outcomes [58]. He argues that checklists help manage complexity and ensure consistency in performing critical tasks. Checklists are simple tools that guide professionals through essential steps in processes, ensuring no critical actions are missed, particularly in high-stakes environments like healthcare.

5.11.12.1   Steps for Checklists

Implementing a checklist in a clinical setting involves several steps [58]. The first step is identifying critical tasks essential to address for a particular process, such as surgery, new patient admission, or very sick patient in the office. Next, develop a clear checklist that includes all identified tasks for the day, ensuring each task is a single, actionable step. At the beginning of the workday review the schedule or patient list, and discuss any priorities with the team. Delegate tasks appropriately. Documentation, prescriptions, triage calls are among the daily tasks deepening on the setting. Make sure to add breaks and time for continuing education or review of a particular disease to gain more understanding. Working through lunch is not productive! With this checklist, the NP can now manage tasks more efficiently using other methods such as the ABCD method.

5.11.13   The ABCD Method

The ABCD method helps NPs systematically evaluate and manage their tasks based on their significance and urgency [59]:

1. NPs assign priorities to each task, categorizing them as A (urgent and necessary), B (important but not urgent), C (urgent but not important), or D (neither urgent nor essential).
2. They set boundaries by determining the time or resources they can allocate to each task.
3. NPs consider the consequences of not completing each task promptly, helping them understand the potential impact on patient care or practice efficiency.

4. Once tasks are completed, NPs mark them as done, allowing for a sense of accomplishment and closure.

Examples

Urgent and important tasks: Responding to a chest pain call requiring immediate triage.

Necessary but not urgent tasks: Conduct scheduled a routine follow-up visit for a patient recovering from pneumonia.

Urgent but not important tasks: Returning calls from patients who need a note for work or waiting to review cholesterol panel.

Neither urgent nor important tasks: non-critical meetings: Attending a continuing education conference.

5.11.14   Getting Things Done

David Allen's "Getting Things Done" (GTD) is a productivity method designed to help people and professionals better manage their tasks and responsibilities [60]. GTD says that minds are more effective at processing information than at storing it. By transferring tasks into a dependable system, individuals can concentrate more on executing tasks rather than remembering them.

GTD revolves around five main steps.

1. Capture
2. Clarify
3. Organize
4. Reflect
5. Engage

The first step, Capture, involves gathering all tasks, ideas, commitments, and information into a reliable system, which could be a notebook or a digital task management tool. The second step, Clarify, involves reviewing these items and deciding on the necessary actions. Items needing action are then further processed, while those not requiring immediate action are deferred. The third step, Organize, focuses on categorizing tasks into lists or calendars, and creating actionable plans. The fourth step, Reflect, involves regularly updating and reviewing the system to keep it current, including daily and weekly check-ins on tasks, projects, and goals. Finally, Engage involves using the organized system to determine which tasks to tackle at any given time, based on context, available time, energy levels, and priorities. This method helps manage workload efficiently and prioritize commitments with a less stressful approach to productivity [60].

5.11.14.1   Application of GTD to the NP
Capture and Clarify

The first step, Capture, involves starting the day by collecting all the information and tasks that need attention [60]. Writing everything down or putting the information into a computer or smartphone to record tasks such as schedule, test results, messages, and prescription refills. This ensures that no task is missed, no matter how small. This next step, clarity, involves reviewing the items to determine the required actions for each. For each patient, the NP decides on the next steps, such as conducting a physical exam, ordering lab tests, or discussing treatment plans. If an item does not require immediate action, categorize it appropriately as trash (not urgent), reference (guidelines), or something to be done later (follow-up calls).

Organize, Reflect, and Engage

In the organizing phase, place tasks and items into appropriate categories such as "to do now," "do later," etc. Use a calendar for time-specific tasks like scheduled appointments or administrative meetings. As one organizes, review and reflection of the list will assess the progress of ongoing goals. For example, quality improvement initiatives will need to be followed. Daily reviews help plan the day effectively, while weekly reviews assess progress on longer-term projects, such as improvement initiatives. Engaging with an organized system to decide what to work on next based on one's time, energy, and priority. This ensures the most important tasks will be addressed but also moving forward.

5.12   Conclusion

Effective time management prevents burnout, particularly in high-stress environments like healthcare. The evolution of time management principles, from early methods like Taylorism to contemporary strategies, underscores the need to balance efficiency with well-being. Initially focused on maximizing productivity through task optimization, time management approaches have evolved to incorporate holistic strategies that address professional and personal well-being.

Implementing modern methodologies such as GTD, utilizing automation tools, and adopting prioritization techniques can significantly enhance productivity while reducing stress. These strategies improve clinical efficiency and patient outcomes and ensure higher patient satisfaction and better overall care. For new NPs, mastering time management is particularly important as they navigate the demanding responsibilities of their initial years in practice.

The challenges posed by the COVID-19 pandemic further underscore the importance of adaptable time management strategies. With increased workloads and shifting practice environments, NPs must remain flexible and resilient. Adopting a holistic approach that incorporates technology, continuous reflection, and adaptable planning helps NPs manage their time effectively while maintaining a sustainable work-life balance. Regular breaks refresh the mind and reduce the risk of mental fatigue, a significant contributor to burnout.

Healthcare organizations should provide ongoing support and resources to help NPs develop and refine their time management skills. This support empowers NPs to deliver high-quality patient care, maintain their well-being, and thrive. Embracing these practices not only enhances productivity during work hours nut also and ensures dedicated time for individual life, contributing to a healthier work-life equilibrium. Ultimately, each NP will find a strategy that works best for them.

Assignment for Time Management

Top of Form

Bottom of Form

Goal: To apply the ABCD method in your practice, demonstrate effective task prioritization, manage time more efficiently, and ensure that critical responsibilities are addressed promptly to deliver high-quality patient care.

Objectives:

1. Apply the ABCD method to effectively prioritize tasks throughout the clinical day.
2. Analyze the potential consequences of delaying tasks.
3. Demonstrate efficient time management.

Case Scenario:

You are a new NP completing a clinical rotation in a primary care practice. Today, you are assigned to work alongside your preceptor, who is a seasoned NP, and you have a full schedule of patient appointments, administrative tasks, and follow-ups to manage. You arrive at 7:30 a.m. and your first patient is at 8:00 a.m.

One of your first patients, Mrs. Messy is a 65-year-old with a past medical history of hypertension and diabetes, is scheduled for a follow-up appointment to review her blood pressures, fingerstick readings, lab results, and medication regimen.

Additionally, you have three new patient appointments booked for today to establish care. There are three acute visits that have a chief

(continued)

(continued)

complaint of chronic cough, dyspnea, and knee pain. You also have several administrative tasks to complete, including reviewing and responding to patient messages in the electronic health record (EHR), updating medication lists, and documenting today's encounters. Two triage calls are waiting, one for chest pain and one for toe pain. There is a form from the billing department to sign and return for recredentialing with an insurance company.

Using the ABCD method, prioritize your tasks for the day, considering the urgency and importance of each, and set realistic boundaries to ensure that tasks are completed within specified timeframes. Consider the possible consequences of task delays and how they may impact patient care. Throughout the day, track the progress and mark tasks as "done" as they are completed to maintain a sense of accomplishment and accountability.

As you navigate through the day, reflect on the effectiveness of your time management strategies and identify areas for improvement. Utilize your preceptor's guidance and feedback to refine your approach and enhance your skills in prioritizing tasks and managing your time as an NP in a primary care setting.

Assign: Begin by listing all tasks for the day and assigning priorities using the ABCD categorization (A for urgent and important, B for important but not urgent, C for urgent but not important, and D for neither urgent nor important).

Boundary: Set specific boundaries for each task, determining the time and resources you can allocate to them. For example, allocate 30 minutes for patient assessments, one hour for chart documentation, and 15 minutes for returning patient calls.

Consequence: Consider the consequences of not completing each task in a timely manner. Reflect on how delays may impact patient care, practice workflow, and overall productivity.

Done: As you complete each task, mark as done to track progress and maintain a sense of accomplishment throughout the day.

Criteria	Excellent (4)	Good (3)	Fair (2)	Needs Improvement (1)
Assignment Completion	All aspects of the ABCD method are thoroughly applied. Tasks are clearly prioritized	Most aspects of the ABCD method are applied, and tasks are prioritized with some clarity	Some aspects of the ABCD method are applied, but tasks may lack clear prioritization	The ABCD method is not effectively applied

(continued)

(continued)

Criteria	Excellent (4)	Good (3)	Fair (2)	Needs Improvement (1)
Boundary Setting	Clear and realistic boundaries are set for each task	Boundaries are set for most tasks, but some may lack specificity or feasibility	Boundaries for tasks are inconsistently set, and some may be unrealistic or overly vague	Boundaries for tasks are not clearly defined or are absent
Consideration of Consequences	Thorough consideration is given to the potential consequences of not completing each task in a timely	Some consideration is given to the consequences of task delays, but it may lack depth	Limited consideration is given to the consequences of task delays, and the impact on patient care	Little to no consideration is given to the consequences of task delays, and the potential impact on patient care

manner, demonstrating insight into the impact on patient care and practice efficiency	or insight into the broader implications	and practice efficiency is not fully addressed	and practice efficiency is overlooked
Task Completion			
All tasks are completed within the specified boundaries	Most tasks are completed within the specified boundaries	Some tasks are completed within the specified boundaries	Few tasks are completed within the specified boundaries

5.13   Legal and Regulatory Constraints

5.13.1   Introduction

In the ever-evolving landscape of healthcare, NPs must continuously keep current with regulatory requirements to provide safe and legal patient care. This section reviews current laws and regulations governing NP practice and strategies for maintaining professional standards. Maintaining integrity and practicing within the legal scope are mandatory for NPs in delivering healthcare. NPs must adhere to their defined scope of practice to ensure patient safety, legal compliance, and professional integrity.

5.13.2   Scope of Practice Definition

The scope of practice for NPs includes the procedures, actions, and processes that they are legally permitted to perform based on their professional license. For example, in states with full practice authority (FPA), NPs can evaluate patients, diagnose conditions, interpret diagnostic tests, and initiate treatment plans independently [61].

5.13.3   Legal Regulations

The legal regulations for NPs in the United States vary by state, as each state has its scope of practice and regulations. However, some general legal considerations apply to NPs nationwide. First, NPs must obtain both an RN license and an advanced practice registered nurse (APRN) license granted by state nursing boards [61]. Additionally, the scope of practice for NPs, which defines their authorized activities and responsibilities, is determined by state law. Some states grant FPA, allowing NPs to practice independently, while others require physician collaboration [61].

5.13.4   Influencing Factors

Several factors, including state laws and regulations, state nursing board rules, and national certification standards, influence the scope of practice for NPs. Each state's Nurse Practice Act outlines specific activities and responsibilities for NPs, impacting their level of autonomy [61]. State nursing boards establish licensure, education, and practice requirements and may also set guidelines for physician collaboration if needed. Moreover, the educational preparation and certification of NPs, typically involving advanced clinical training and degrees, influence their breadth of knowledge and skills, thereby affecting their scope of practice [62].

5.13.5   State Regulations and Examples

State regulations for NPs vary significantly across the United States, impacting their scope of practice. For example, in California, NPs must work collaboratively with a physician. This agreement mandates specific protocols and oversight by the physician, limiting the NP's autonomy [63]. In contrast, Arizona grants NPs FPA, allowing them to operate independently without physician oversight. This level of independence enables NPs in Arizona to diagnose, treat, and prescribe medications independently [64].

Texas represents a more restrictive environment for NPs. They must have a collaborative agreement with a physician and are subject to specific requirements regarding the delegation of prescriptive authority. This collaboration must include regular meetings and reviews of the NP's practice [65]. Conversely, NPs enjoy FPA in Oregon, similar to Arizona. They can provide comprehensive care independently, enhancing access to healthcare services, especially in rural and underserved areas [66].

In Georgia, the scope of practice for NPs requires a required collaborative agreement with a physician. The agreement specifies the medical acts and prescriptive authority delegated to the NP, ensuring physician oversight is maintained [67]. Meanwhile, Colorado allows NPs to practice independently after completing a provisional period under physician supervision, thus granting FPA after demonstrating competency [68].

Given these variations, it is crucial for NPs to regularly review their state's Nurse Practice Act and any updates to stay compliant with current regulations. Understanding the specific requirements and limitations in their state ensures that NPs practice within the legal framework and maintain the highest standards of patient care.

5.13.6   Practice and Prescriptive Authority

The 36th Annual Advanced Practice Registered Nurses (APRN) Legislative Update provided an overview of the current state of practice and prescriptive authority in various states [69]. In recent years, various states have made significant advancements in granting NPs greater autonomy, particularly around prescriptive authority.

According to this update, several states have implemented legislative changes to expand NPs' scope of practice and prescribing rights. For instance, Arizona now allows healthcare providers to dispense a 12-hour supply of opioid medication upon discharge if no 24-hour pharmacy is nearby. Utah eliminated the Transition to Practice (TTP) period requirement for prescribing Schedule II controlled substances, making it the 28th state to authorize FPA. In Illinois, APRNs with FPA can prescribe up to a 120-day supply of benzodiazepines without a physician consultation, though continued prescriptions require a physician's input. Kentucky improved controlled substance (CS) prescriptive authority, allowing APRNs with four years of practice under a collaborative agreement to gain limited autonomous prescriptive rights [69].

5.13.7   Malpractice Insurance

NPs must carefully consider whether to rely solely on employer-provided professional liability insurance or obtain their own individual policies [70]. While many healthcare organizations, hospitals, and clinics provide liability insurance for their employees, this coverage often has limitations and exclusions that can leave NPs vulnerable in certain situations. Employer-provided liability insurance generally covers NPs for claims arising from their professional duties performed within the scope of their employment. However, this coverage may not extend to activities outside their primary job, such as moonlighting, volunteer work, or other part-time jobs. Additionally, employer policies tend to prioritize the organization's interests, which may not always align with the NP's interests during a claim [70].

Obtaining an individual liability insurance policy offers several advantages. These policies provide comprehensive coverage, including protection for work outside the primary employment. Individual policies also allow NPs to have legal representation, which can be crucial if there is a conflict of interest between the NP and their employer. Moreover, personal policies often include additional benefits such as reputation protection, which are not typically covered by employer policies [71].

Given these factors, it is generally recommended that NPs carry their own professional liability insurance in addition to any employer-provided coverage. This ensures they have continuous and comprehensive protection, regardless of employment changes or specific exclusions in the employer's policy. Individual insurance provides peace of mind and safeguards NPs against the financial and professional risks of malpractice claims.

5.13.8   Collaboration and Referrals

Effective interprofessional collaboration and robust referral systems are crucial for comprehensive patient care in nursing practice. Collaboration involves working closely with specialists to ensure that patients receive holistic care while staying within the NP's scope of practice. For instance, an NP might collaborate with a pulmonologist to manage a patient with complex respiratory issues, ensuring the patient benefits from specialized expertise. In cases of cardiovascular diseases, NPs often work alongside cardiologists to optimize medication management, perform necessary diagnostics like echocardiograms, and provide comprehensive care, thereby enhancing patient outcomes [70].

Referral systems are equally important, allowing NPs to direct patients to the appropriate level of care efficiently. For example, if an NP suspects a cancer diagnosis in a patient, they should promptly refer the patient to an oncologist for further evaluation and treatment. This ensures timely intervention for the best possible outcomes in cancer care. Similarly, when an NP identifies a patient requiring surgical intervention, such as acute appendicitis, prompt referral to a general surgeon is essential to prevent complications. These practices enhance patient outcomes and ensure timely and appropriate interventions, reinforcing the importance of collaboration and referral systems in advanced nursing practice [72].

5.13.9 Legislation

New NPs must stay current with laws and regulations to ensure they provide safe and legally compliant care. This involves awareness of emerging and changing regulations that may impact their practice. To stay informed, NPs should utilize resources that update them on how these changes affect their work. For example, being active in professional organizations such as the American Association of Nurse Practitioners (AANP) or specialty-specific groups can provide valuable access to updates, education webinars, and newsletters focused on regulatory changes [73]. Engaging with one's state NP organizations can help the NP stay abreast of local regulations and practice standards. The NP must keep updated on emerging policies and guidelines that may affect their practice, including changes related to telehealth, healthcare reform, and public health emergencies.

5.13.9.1 Pronouncing Death Example

NPs can pronounce death in several states, with specific regulations varying by location. States where NPs can pronounce death include California, New York, Texas, Oregon, Vermont, Maine, Virginia, Washington, Hawaii, Maryland, and New Jersey. In some states, this authority extends to signing death certificates and is often conditional upon adhering to specific guidelines and protocols [73]. For example, in Texas, NPs can pronounce death, particularly in hospice settings, while in New York and Oregon, they are also authorized to sign death certificates. What if the NP is working in a hospital and asked to pronounce death? Are they allowed to in that state? It is essential for NPs to stay informed about their state's specific laws and regulations, as these can change. For the most current information, NPs should refer to their state's nursing board or professional organizations like the AANP.

Legislation Assignment

Goal: To enhance the understanding of current legislative trends affecting NPs and their impact on practice.

Objectives:

1. Analyze recent legislation affecting NPs.
2. Evaluate the potential effects of a selected bill on NPs and patients.

Instructions: For this exercise, visit www.congress. gov and search for "Nurse Practitioner Legislation." Review recent bills and their last actions to understand current legislative trends and impacts on NP practice. This assignment can be done online or in person.

Discussion Assignment:

1. Pick a Bill that affects NP's.
2. Identify and tell the group what it is about any action on this bill lately?
3. How would the passing of this bill affect NPs and patients?
4. Identify who your local representatives are and why contacting them would matter.

Criteria	Excellent (4pts)	Proficient (3 pts)	Needs Improvement (2pts)	Unsatisfactory (1 pt)
Bill Selection	Clearly identifies a relevant bill and explains its key points	Identifies a relevant bill and gives a basic explanation	Identifies a bill but explanation is unclear or incomplete	Does not identify a relevant bill or explanation is incorrect
Impact Analysis	Thoroughly explains how the bill affects NPs and patients	Explains how the bill affects NPs and patients with some detail	Provides a brief or unclear explanation of the bill's impact	Does not explain the bill's impact or is incorrect
Representative Identification	Correctly names local representatives and explains why contacting them matters	Names local representatives and gives a basic reason to contact them	Names representatives but does not explain why contacting them matters	Does not name representatives or explanation is unclear

5.14   Conclusion

In the healthcare field, legislative changes continually shape the practice of NPs and their role in patient care. Understanding and staying current with these evolving regulations should be a priority for NPs to ensure compliance and maintain high standards of care. Each legislative development can significantly impact how NPs operate and interact with other healthcare providers, from scope of practice variations to prescriptive authority shifts. By actively engaging with professional organizations, and regularly reviewing relevant legislation, NPs can navigate these complexities successfully.

References

1. Benner, P. (1984). *From Novice to Expert: Excellence and Power in Clinical Nursing Practice*. Menlo Park: Addison-Wesley.
2. Kolb, D.A. (1984). *Experiential Learning: Experience as the Source of Learning and Development*. Englewood Cliffs: Prentice Hall.
3. Clance, P.R. and Imes, S.A. (1978). The impostor phenomenon in high achieving women: dynamics and therapeutic intervention. *Psychother Theory Res Pract.* 15 (3): 241–247. https://doi.org/10.1037/h0086006.
4. UCLA Health (2023). Imposter syndrome among medical students. https://www.uclahealth.org/imposter-syndrome (accessed 22 August 2024).
5. Henning, K., Ey, S., and Shaw, D. (1998). Perfectionism, the impostor phenomenon, and psychological adjustment in medical, dental, nursing and pharmacy students. *Med. Educ.* 32 (5): 456–464.
6. McGregor, L.N., Gee, D.E., and Posey, K.E. (2008). I feel like a fraud, and it depresses me: the relation between the impostor phenomenon and depression. *Soc. Behav. Personal.* 36 (1): 43–48.

7. Villwock, J.A., Sobin, L.B., Koester, L.A., and Harris, T.M. (2016). Impostor syndrome and burnout among American medical students: a pilot study. *Int. J. Med. Educ.* 7: 364–369.

8. Bernard, N.S., Dollinger, S.J., and Ramaniah, N.V. (2002). Applying the big five personality factors to the impostor phenomenon. *J. Pers. Assess.* 78 (2): 321–333.

9. Neureiter, M. and Traut-Mattausch, E. (2016). Inspecting the potential link between the imposter phenomenon and maladaptive perfectionism. *Personal. Individ. Differ.* 102: 93–98.

10. Gonzalez, C.M. and Lypson, M.L. (2014). Microaggressions: clarification, delineation, and implications for medical education. *Acad. Med.* 89 (6): 854–860.

11. Hutchins, H.M. and Rainbolt, H. (2016). What triggers impostor phenomenon among academic faculty? A critical incident study exploring antecedents, coping, and development opportunities. *Hum. Resour. Dev. Int.* 20 (3): 194–214.

12. Kleina, J. and Gribbins, A. (2021). Mentoring new graduate nurse practitioners to decrease transition-to-practice stress and increase retention. *J. Nurse Pract.* 17 (2): 216–219.

13. Peng, Y., Xiao, S.W., Tu, H. et al. (2022). The impostor phenomenon among nursing students and nurses: a scoping review. *Front. Psychol.* 13: 809031. `https://doi.org/10.3389/fpsyg.2022.809031`. PMID: 35356345; PMCID: PMC8959846.

14. Bravata, D.M., Watts, S.A., Keefer, A.L. et al. (2020). Prevalence, predictors, and treatment of impostor syndrome: a systematic review. *J. Gen. Intern. Med.* 35 (4): 1252–1275.

15. Speight, C., Firnhaber, G., Scott, E.S., and Wei, H. (2019). Strategies to promote the professional transition of new graduate nurse practitioners: a systematic review. *Nurs. Forum* 54 (4): 557–564. `https://doi.org/10.1111/nuf.12370`. Epub 2019 Jul 24. PMID: 31339178.

16. Erickson, C.E., Steen, D., French-Baker, K., and Ash, L. (2021). Establishing organizational support for nurse practitioner/physician assistant transition to practice programs. *J. Nurse Pract.* 17 (4): 485–488.

17. Ortiz Pate, K., Muñoz, P., and Young, C. (2022). Successful strategies for onboarding nurse practitioners and physician assistants in primary care. *J. Nurse Pract.* 18 (6): 567–573.

18. Haney, J.L., Birkholz, L., and Rutledge, C. (2018). A workshop for addressing the impact of the imposter syndrome on clinical nurse specialists. *Clin. Nurse Spec.* 32 (3): 189–194. https:// doi.org/10.1097/NUR.0000000000000386.

19. Mullins, L.J. (2018). Peer support: mutual support can help new nurse practitioners. *Nurse Pract.* 43 (4): 9–12.

20. Joint Commission (2021). The importance of credentialing and privileging. https://www.jointcommission.org (accessed 21 August 2024.

21. National Committee for Quality Assurance (2024). Accreditation standards. www.ncqa.org (accessed 23 June 2024).

22. Medical Group Management Association (2024). Credentialing guidelines. www.mgma.com (accessed 21 September 2024).

23. Vance, C. and Gildemeister, S. (2020). Credentialing and competency verification for nurse practitioners: a comprehensive approach. *J. Am. Assoc. Nurse Pract.* 32 (4): 247–254. https:// doi.org/10.1097/JXX.0000000000000178.

24. Kovner, C.T., Djukic, M., and Fatehi, F. (2020). A review of competency-based training for nurse practitioners: ensuring safe and effective patient care. *J. Nurs. Scholarsh.* 52 (6): 676–684. https://doi.org/10.1111/jonm.12963.

25. Eustache, S., Schwenk, S.T., and Hinojosa, M.S. (2023). The process of obtaining a DEA number for nurse practitioners: a comprehensive guide. *J. Am. Assoc. Nurse Pract.* 35 (5): 234–240. https://doi.org/10.1097/JXX.0000000000000289.

26. American Academy of Family Physicians (2023). New DEA training requirement: who has to do it, and how to get it done. https:// www.aafp.org/pubs/fpm/blogs/inpractice/entry/new-dea-requirement.html (accessed 22 September 2024).

27. Elite, N.P. (2023). How to meet the DEA's one-time training requirement for substance use disorders. https://www.elitenp.com/resources/dea-training-requirements. (accessed 21 July 2024).

28. Centers for Medicare & Medicaid Services (2024). National Plan and Provider Enumeration System (NPPES) for NPI. https://nppes.cms.hhs.gov/NPPES/Welcome.do (accessed 09 September 2024).

29. Anderson, G.F. (2022). The impact of the National Provider Identifier on healthcare administration. *Health Aff.*

(Millwood) 41 (7): 102–110. https://doi.org/10.1377/hlthaff.2022.00056.

30. Academy of Nurse Practitioners (2023). Understanding NPI and its importance for nurse practitioners. https://www.aanp.org/education/npi. (accessed 20 September 2024).

31. Beardsley, A. and Jones, J. (2020). Introduction to privileges: credentialing versus privileging and CMS requirements. Health-Stream. www.healthstream.com (accessed 08 May 2020).

32. Wang, J., Zhang, C., and Liu, X. (2022). Ongoing professional development for nurse practitioners: recredentialing, CEUs, and recertification. *Nurse Educ.* 47 (5): 234–240. https://doi.org/10.1097/NNE.0000000000001158.

33. Goh, S.L., Lewis, A., and Anthony, A.S. (2021). The importance of recredentialing for nurse practitioners: maintaining competence and professional standards. *J. Nurs. Regul.* 12 (3): 45–50. https://doi.org/10.1016/j.jnr.2021.07.003.

34. National Association of Credential Evaluation Services (2023). Steps for credentialing nurses and physician assistants in a hospital setting. https://www.naces.org/credentialing-nurses-and-pas-hospital (accessed 23 June 2024).

35. Centers for Medicare & Medicaid Services (2023). Provider enrollment and certification. www.cms.gov (accessed 09 May 2024).

36. Council for Affordable Quality Healthcare (2023). Credentialing and recredentialing. https://www.caqh.org/solutions/caqh-proview (accessed 08 July 2024).

37. UnitedHealthcare (2023). Credentialing plan and process. UnitedHealthcare. https://www.uhcprovider.com/content/dam/provider/docs/public/resources/join-network/Credentialing-Plan.pdf (accessed 08 July 2024).

38. American Academy of Nurse Practitioners (2023). Billing and coding for nurse practitioners. AANP https://www.aanp.org/practice/practice-management/business-resources-for-nurse-practitioners (accessed 20 September 2024).

39. Centers for Medicare & Medicaid Services (2022). Nurse practitioner services. CMS https://www.cms.gov/medicare/payment/fee-schedules/physician-fee-schedule/advanced-practice-nonphysician-practitioners/advanced-practice-registered-nurses-aprns (accessed 09 September 2024).

40. Claessens, B.J., Eerde, W.V., Rutte, C.G., and Roe, R.A. (2007). A review of the time management literature. *Pers. Rev.* 36 (2): 255–276.
41. Ariella, S. (2023). 23 opportune time management statistics [2023]: facts, data, and trends. *Zippia* (14 November 2022). https://www.zippia.com/advice/time-management-statistics.
42. Taylor, H. (2019). History of time management. In: *Taylor in Time*. Retrieved July 6, 2024, from https://www.taylorintime.com/history-of-time-management.
43. Aeon, B. and Aguinis, H. (2017). It's about time: new perspectives and insights on time management. *Acad. Manag. Perspect.* 31 (4): 309–330. https://doi.org/10.5465/amp.2016.0166.
44. Aeon, B., Faber, A., and Panaccio, A. (2021). Does time management work? A meta-analysis. *PLoS One* 16 (1): https://doi.org/10.1371/journal.pone.0245066.
45. Addis, B.A., Gelaw, Y.M., Eyowas, F.A. et al. (2023). "Time wasted by health professionals is time not invested in patients": time management practice and associated factors among health professionals at public hospitals in Bahir Dar, Ethiopia: a multicenter mixed method study. *Front. Public Health* 11: 1159275. https://doi.org/10.3389/fpubh.2023.1159275. PMID: 37546322; PMCID: PMC10403234.
46. Boulding, W., Glickman, S.W., Manary, M.P. et al. (2011). Relationship between patient satisfaction with inpatient care and HCAHPS scores. *Health Serv. Res.* 46 (1): 62–83. https://doi.org/10.1111/j.1475-6773.2010.01199.x.
47. Labrague, L.J., McEnroe-Petitte, D.M., Leocadio, M.C. et al. (2018). Stress and ways of coping among nurse practitioners: a systematic review. *Int. J. Nurs. Stud.* 80: 16–24. https://doi.org/10.1016/j.ijnurstu.2017.12.003.
48. Doran, D.M., Hirdes, J.P., and McGilton, K.S. (2020). The impact of evidence-based guidelines on the quality of care for patients with chronic conditions. *J. Nurs. Care Qual.* 35 (3): 233–240. https://doi.org/10.1097/NCQ.0000000000000440.
49. Monaghesh, E. and Hajizadeh, A. (2020). The role of telehealth during COVID-19 outbreak: a systematic review based on current evidence. *BMC Public Health* 20: 1193. https://doi.org/10.1186/s12889-020-09301-4.

50. Gallup (2021). State of the global workplace. `https://www.gallup.com/workplace/284180/state-global-workplace-2021.aspx` (accessed 08 October 2024).

51. Calendly (2021). The ultimate guide to online appointment booking and scheduling software. `https://calendly.com/blog/online-appointment-booking-scheduling-software` (accessed 09 October 2024).

52. Bates, D.W., Kuperman, G.J., Wang, S. et al. (2003). Ten commandments for effective clinical decision support: making the practice of evidence-based medicine a reality. *J. Am. Med. Inform. Assoc.* 10 (6): 523–530. `https://doi.org/10.1197/jamia.M1370`.

53. Zapier (2020). The ultimate guide to workflow automation. `https://zapier.com/blog/automation` (accessed 10 October 2024).

54. Lee-Yoon, A. and Whillans, A.V. (2019). Making seconds count: when valuing time promotes subjective well-being. *Curr. Opin. Psychol.* 26: 54–57. `https://doi.org/10.1016/j.copsyc.2018.05.002`.

55. Holiday, R. and Hanselman, S. (2016). *The Daily Stoic: 366 Meditations on Wisdom, Perseverance, and the Art of Living.* New York: Portfolio.

56. Zhu, M., Yang, Y., and Hsee, C.K. (2018). The mere urgency effect. *J. Consum. Res.* 45 (3): 673–690. `https://doi.org/10.1093/jcr/ucy008`.

57. Harvard Business Review (2020). Time management is about more than life hacks. `https://hbr.org/2020/01/time-management-is-about-more-than-life-hacks`. (accessed 08 July 2024).

58. Gawande, A. (2009). *The Checklist Manifesto: How to Get Things Right.* New York: Metropolitan Books.

59. Covey, S.R. (2013). *The 7 Habits of Highly Effective People: Powerful Lessons in Personal Change.* New York: Simon & Schuster.

60. Allen, D. (2001). *Getting Things Done: The Art of Stress-Free Productivity.* New York: Penguin Books.

61. National Council of State Boards of Nursing (NCSBN) (2022). Scope of practice decision-making framework. `https://www.ncsbn.org/nursing-regulation/practice/decision-making-framework.page` (accessed 20 July 2024).

62. Phillips, S.J. (2021). 33rd annual APRN legislative update: improvements in practice environment for nurse practitioners. *Nurse Pract.* 46 (1): 22–46.

63. California Board of Registered Nursing (2023). Nurse practitioner practice requirements. www.rn.ca.gov (accessed 01 September 2024).

64. Arizona State Board of Nursing (2023). Nurse practitioner scope of practice. www.azbn.gov (accessed 20 August 2024).

65. Texas Board of Nursing (2023). Advanced practice registered nurse (APRN) practice. https://www.bon.texas.gov (accessed 20 August 2024).

66. Oregon State Board of Nursing (2023). Nurse practitioner practice and regulation. https://www.oregon.gov/osbn (accessed 20 August 2024).

67. Georgia Board of Nursing (2023). Nurse practitioner practice regulations 2023. https://sos.ga.gov/index.php/licensing/plb/45 (accessed 20 August 2024).

68. Colorado Board of Nursing (2023). Advanced practice registered nurse (APRN) requirements 2023. https://dpo.colorado.gov/Nursing (accessed 20 August 2024).

69. Phillips, S.J. (2024). 36th annual APRN legislative update: improving practice scope and authority, one state at a time. *Nurse Pract.* 49 (1): 21–31. Available from: www.tnpj.com.

70. American Association of Nurse Practitioners (2022). Malpractice insurance and nurse practitioners: Understanding your liability coverage. https://storage.aanp.org/www/documents/research/Malpractice-Insurance_FINAL.pdf (accessed 20 June 2024).

71. Berxi (2023). Why nurse practitioners need malpractice insurance. https://www.berxi.com/resources/articles/why-nurse-practitioners-need-malpractice-insurance (accessed 21 June 2024).

72. American Nurses Association (2015). *Nursing: Scope and Standards of Practice*, 3e. Silver Spring, MD: Nursesbooks.org.

73. American Association of Nurse Practitioners (2020). NP fact sheet. https://www.aanp.org/about/all-about-nps/np-fact-sheet (accessed 20 June 2024).

Chapter 6

Patient-Centered Care

Sara L. Gleasman-DeSimone PhD, ANP-C
Le Moyne College, Graduate Nursing Department, Syracuse, NY, USA

A Nurse Practitioner's Insight: Empathy and Trust in Patient-Centered Care
Therese Brown-Mahoney, MSN, CNM, NP
Le Moyne College, Graduate Nursing Department, Syracuse, NY, USA

Professional Practice Guided by Evidence
Gina Myers, PhD, RN
Le Moyne College, Graduate Nursing Department, Syracuse, NY, USA

Nurse Practitioner: Transition Guide, First Edition. Sara L. Gleasman-DeSimone.
© 2025 John Wiley & Sons, Inc. Published 2025 by John Wiley & Sons, Inc.

Chapter Highlights

Empathy
Self-Efficacy
Therapeutic Communication
Motivational Interviewing
Professional Practice Guided by Evidence
Ethical Principles
Patient Education
Cultural Competence
Diversity, Equity, and Inclusion

6.1   Introduction

Nurse practitioners (NPs) are committed to providing patient-centered care that prioritizes the unique needs, values, and preferences of each individual in every encounter. This chapter will explore the key components of patient-centered care, including the development of therapeutic relationships and the delivery of comprehensive patient education to empower patients. It will also address communication strategies that foster trust and understanding, along with techniques for managing challenging patient interactions. Ethical considerations, such as respecting patient autonomy and promoting diversity, equity, and inclusion (DEI), are integral to ensuring all patients feel respected, heard, and valued. Equally important is the application of evidence-based practice in guiding clinical decisions, a cornerstone of the NP's professional role. This chapter will equip new NPs with the essential tools to navigate complex situations and thrive in their practice.

Chapter Objectives and Mapping to 2021 AACN Masters Essentials

1. Describe the principles of patient-centered care and how they guide clinical practice. Domain 2: Person-Centered Care. Domain 1: Knowledge for Nursing Practice.

2. Analyze the role of therapeutic communication techniques in building trust and enhancing patient–provider relationships. Domain 6: Interprofessional Partnerships. Domain 7: Systems-Based Practice.

3. Apply motivational interviewing and empathy to manage patient interactions effectively. Domain 2: Person-Centered Care. Domain 4: Nursing Judgment.

4. Evaluate the ethical dimensions of patient care. Domain 8: Information and Healthcare Technologies. Domain 9: Professionalism.

5. Evaluate the quality and relevance of clinical practice guidelines and systematic reviews to integrate evidence-based practice into patient-centered care. Domain 3: Scholarship for the Nursing Discipline. Domain 8: Clinical Judgment and Evidence-Based Care.

6. Discuss a personalized care plan that integrates patient preferences, cultural considerations, and collaborative problem-solving. Domain 5: Quality and Safety. Domain 6: Domain 2: Person-Centered Care.

6.2 Patient Communication

Patient-centered care is rooted in establishing a partnership between the healthcare provider and the patient. This includes a focus on the individual's unique needs, preferences, and values, which are integral to providing personalized care [1]. During the first year of practice, NPs lay the foundation for patient-centered care. They do this by honing their communication skills and fostering a patient–provider relationship built on trust and collaboration. Effective communication involves active listening, empathy, and clear, understandable dialogue. By acknowledging and understanding the patient's perspective, NPs can tailor their approach to meet unique individual requirements [2]. This empathetic connection serves as the foundation of a therapeutic relationship, significantly enhancing patient satisfaction and health outcomes [3].

6.2.1 Patient Communication and Outcomes

Effective communication between providers and patients plays a fundamental role in improving health outcomes. Effective communication helps reduce patient anxiety, fosters trust, and promotes patient understanding and agreement on the plan of care [2]. This leads to better adherence to treatment and improved self-care, both of which contribute to long-term health benefits. Furthermore, effective communication can enhance access to care, empower patients, and improve decision-making, all of which further boost patient health. Patient-centered communication is also correlated with better disease management and lower anxiety levels. Future research should continue to explore specific pathways that link communication to health outcomes to develop targeted strategies for improving patient care [2]. In addition to improved disease management and reduced anxiety, effective communication plays a critical role in building trust between patients and providers.

6.2.1.1 Trust and Perceptions

Trust, as a key outcome of patient-centered communication, is foundational to patients' overall perceptions of care quality and their willingness to adhere to treatment plans. Patient-centered communication influences two key outcomes: patients' trust in their healthcare providers and their perceptions of healthcare quality [4]. Trust was identified as a more immediate result of communication, while perceptions of healthcare quality were considered a longer-term outcome, both contributing to overall health. Trust also served as a bridge between communication and healthcare quality, with its impact growing as patients experienced more frequent hospital visits. This underscores the significance of effective communication in enhancing patient trust and overall healthcare experiences.

6.2.1.2 Cost

In addition to building trust, patient-centered care has been showed to impact healthcare costs. Bertakis and Azari (2011) examined patient-centered care through an analysis system called the Davis Observation Code (DOC) [5]. The DOC is an observational tool used to analyze and categorize behaviors during medical visits between healthcare providers and patients. Their findings indicated that patient-centered interactions were associated with lower overall healthcare costs, particularly by contributing to the reduction of diagnostic tests and hospitalizations. The patient-centered care approach encompassed behaviors such as shared decision-making, addressing psychosocial aspects, and discussing family dynamics. Although patient-centered care was not directly linked to higher patient satisfaction during initial visits, the study concluded that it significantly contributed to reducing medical costs [5]. This approach emphasized understanding patients in the context of their own lives and empowering them to manage their health more effectively.

6.2.2 Psychological Principles of Patient-Centered Care

6.2.2.1 Empathy

Empathy is a fundamental component of patient-centered care, encompassing both the emotional and cognitive dimensions of understanding a patient's feelings [6]. Affective empathy involves sharing the patient's emotions, while cognitive empathy requires putting oneself in the patient's shoes. Empathic communication, through understanding and sharing feelings, ultimately enhances patient satisfaction, reduces medical errors, and lowers legal risks. Overall, this is a tool for enhancing patient outcomes and fostering trust in healthcare settings [6]. Patients want their providers to listen and truly understand them. Simple strategies that emphasize empathy and improve communication methods can help patients feel more valued and comfortable in public healthcare environments [6]. Building on the importance of empathy, the following insights demonstrate how NPs can establish trust in even the most time-constrained clinical environments.

6.2.2.2   A Nurse Practitioner's Insight: Empathy and Trust in Patient-Centered Care

By, Therese Brown-Mahoney, MSN, CNM, NP

How can you begin to create a harmonious, positive, trusting relationship with a patient within the time constraints of a full schedule of patients? You have 15 minutes to see a patient and you are already half-an-hour-behind schedule. It is imperative that a patient feels understood for you to connect. Despite the ticking clock, take a deep breath and be prepared to enter your patients' world as it exists for them at this period.

It is ideal if you can meet a patient for the first time while they are dressed. It allows them to feel less vulnerable. The reality is that the medical assistant or nurse you work with may have already taken a history, vital signs, and had the patient get undressed. Get the basic information from your team before you enter the room. Patients feel unheard when they have already described their problem to the medical assistant or nurse, and you as the NP go in and expect the patient to repeat it all.

First, enter the room, introduce yourself, put your chart, laptop, or computer aside, and SIT DOWN. Maintain eye contact. Ask some easy questions first, i.e., for a teenager coming in for her first visit, ask about schooling and extra-curricular activities.

Now you are ready to connect with empathy. LISTEN WITH INTENT and believe that this is their experience, unique to them. If a teenager is coming in to talk about her heavy and painful menses (even though it may seem to be a normal menses), this is what the teenager is experiencing. It is her perception or perhaps an excuse to talk about their sexuality and desire for contraception.

Define the problem. Going back to our teenager, repeat what she is saying: If I am hearing you right, the heavy and painful menses you are experiencing are interfering with your school day, sports life, or social life.

Now you are ready for the physical examination. Always describe exactly what you are doing and why. Always ask for permission for any kind of uncovering any body part and for permission for any kind of touch. For example, I will need to palpate your abdomen (palpate means to push on your belly with firm pressure). Define terms in an easy-to-understand language.

After your examination, and the patient is dressed, it is time for collaborative problem-solving. You may be ready to dig a little deeper at this point and ask some of the more uncomfortable questions in the name of choosing the right strategy together to solve the problem. Now you can ask about sexual behavior that can also be addressed with the same method used to help with heavy and painful menses.

In a nutshell, connect with empathy, define the problem, and collaborate to solve it.

6.2.2.3 Self-Efficacy

Self-efficacy refers to a person's belief in their ability to manage and succeed in different situations [7]. This belief significantly influences behavior, shaping how individuals think, feel, and act in various circumstances. People with high self-efficacy are more likely to take on challenges with confidence and actively engage in tasks, often finding satisfaction in the process. Even when setbacks occur, they tend to recover quickly and experience less stress, which helps them persist and remain resilient. On the other hand, individuals with low self-efficacy may view challenges as threats and focus on their limitations, leading to avoidance behaviors. This mindset can lead to lower commitment to goals, a tendency to give up when faced with difficulties, and increased susceptibility to stress and depression. In this way, self-efficacy serves as a key determinant of how people navigate and respond to life's demands.

Building Self-Efficacy

Building self-efficacy involves four key factors: mastery experiences, social modeling, social persuasion, and the influence of emotional and physiological states [7]. These factors shape an individual's belief in their effectiveness, which in turn affects how they cope and handle challenges. Mastery experiences, such as successfully overcoming challenges, are the most effective way to build self-efficacy. Each success enhances confidence and prepares individuals to handle future obstacles more effectively. For instance, completing a difficult project can boost one's confidence in tackling similar tasks in the future. Social modeling, or observing others who succeed, reinforces the belief that similar success is possible. For example, seeing a peer excel in a particular area can inspire the belief that one can do the same. Social persuasion, through encouragement and positive feedback from others, can further strengthen self-efficacy [7]. Supportive words from a mentor, for example, can increase determination and help individuals focus on their strengths rather than their doubts. Finally, emotional and physiological states play a role in self-efficacy. A positive mood can lead to a more favorable assessment of one's abilities, while stress or anxiety can undermine confidence and reduce the likelihood of taking on challenges.

The Role of Self-Efficacy in Shaping Behavior and Outcomes

Self-efficacy plays a crucial role in shaping behavior by influencing how individuals approach challenges, set goals, and manage their emotions [7]. Those with high self-efficacy tend to think positively, set ambitious goals, and remain committed to achieving them, resulting in more effective coping strategies and better performance outcomes. Their confidence allows them to manage emotions more effectively, focusing on overcoming obstacles rather than becoming overwhelmed. This persistence leads to positive outcomes, such as greater achievement, resilience, and personal growth [8]. Conversely, individuals with low self-efficacy often see challenges as overwhelming, leading to avoidance behaviors that limit their personal and professional growth.

In healthcare, higher self-efficacy is linked to improved health outcomes, including better coping strategies and greater resilience in the face of illness. For instance, Li et al. (2024) investigated the role of self-efficacy in the relationship between body image and sleep quality among breast cancer patients. Using tools like the General Perceived Self-Efficacy Scale and the Body Image Scale, the study found that patients with higher self-efficacy experienced better sleep quality. These patients were more capable of managing emotional stress related to body image following breast cancer treatment, leading to fewer sleep disturbances. Patients with high self-efficacy were also more successful in regulating their emotions and adopting positive coping strategies, contributing to overall emotional well-being. This suggests that interventions aimed at enhancing self-efficacy, such as cognitive behavioral therapy, could improve both emotional and physical health outcomes in breast cancer patients. By fostering self-efficacy, healthcare providers can help patients manage body image concerns more effectively, ultimately leading to improved overall health outcomes [8].

Application of Self-Efficacy

In clinical practice, self-efficacy is applied as a key factor that influences a patient's ability to engage in and main health-promoting behaviors. It refers to the confidence individuals have in their ability to perform specific actions in various situations [9]. NPs play a crucial role in enhancing self-efficacy by tailoring education to the patient's level of understanding, thereby empowering them to make informed decisions about their health. For instance, breaking down complex changes into manageable steps and celebrating small successes can significantly boost a patient's confidence in their ability to implement those changes. Additionally, the presence or absence of social support can greatly influence self-efficacy. When social support is lacking, a patient's self-efficacy may decrease, leading to a lower likelihood of adopting and maintaining recommended behaviors [9]. Patients who lack confidence in their ability to manage their care often avoid health-promoting activities, whereas those with robust support systems are more likely to adhere to their care plans, particularly in areas such as physical activity. This highlights the intertwined roles of self-efficacy and social support in helping patients manage their health effectively [9].

6.2.2.4 Managing Challenging Patient Interactions

In NP school, students are taught to adhere to standard guidelines for managing conditions such as hypertension or asthma. While these standards of care are important to follow, what can the NP do when a patient refuses to comply or doesn't understand or disagrees with recommendations? NPs inevitably face challenging patient interactions. Whether these challenges arise from non-compliance, cultural differences, or communication barriers, successfully navigating them requires a careful balance of sensitivity, professionalism, and adaptability.

When encountering challenging patients, NPs must adopt a patient-centered approach that emphasizes patience, empathy, and a non-judgmental attitude. Understanding the underlying issues that may be driving a patient's behavior, allows practitioners to tailor their interactions to meet the unique needs of individuals [10]. This not only strengthens the patient–provider relationship but also promotes better health outcomes. To de-escalate tensions effectively, maintaining a calm and peaceful demeanor is imperative as it sets a positive tone for the interaction. Acknowledging the patient's emotions, which helps them feel validated, can diffuse anger and frustration. Active listening, which involves giving the patient one's full attention and reflecting on their concerns will ensure that they feel understood. Additionally, maintaining open and non-threatening body language further helps ease tensions [11]. Allowing patients space to vent their frustrations without interruption, combined with showing empathy and understanding, can significantly reduce conflict. Once the situation is de-escalated, collaborating with the patient to find solutions that meet their needs while ensuring clinical safety is vital. When necessary, setting clear boundaries can prevent further escalation. These strategies are widely recommended in healthcare settings to ensure both patient and staff safety, ultimately leading to improved patient outcomes [12].

6.2.2.5 Enhancing Patient Engagement Through Therapeutic Communication

In the realm of patient-centered care, effective therapeutic communication is essential for building strong patient–provider relationships and promoting positive health outcomes. Utilizing various communication techniques allows NPs to understand patients' needs better, foster trust, and encourage active participation in their care. For example, giving recognition and acknowledging patients' achievements, no matter how small, also contribute to a supportive and motivating healthcare environment. By incorporating patients' personal goals and successes into the care plan, NPs create a more holistic and patient-driven approach [13]. The following table offers some common therapeutic communication techniques with examples that illustrate their application in NP practice.

Therapeutic Communication Technique	Description	Examples
Active Listening	Fully concentrating, understanding, and responding to the patient	"Eye contact. Face the patient. Nodding to show one is listening."
Empathy	Understanding and sharing the feelings of the patient	"That sounds really difficult. I can understand why you're feeling upset."

(continued)

Therapeutic Communication Technique	Description	Examples
Clarification	Asking for more information to ensure understanding	"Can you explain what you mean when you say you're feeling overwhelmed?"
Open-Ended Questions	Encouraging patients to express themselves in more detail	"How do you feel about using this inhaler consistently?"
Reflection	Echoing back the patient's feelings or thoughts to show understanding	"It sounds like you're feeling frustrated because of the delays."
Summarization	Recapping what the patient has said to confirm understanding	"So, what I hear you saying is that you're concerned about the side effects."
Validation	Affirming the patient's feelings and experiences	"It makes sense that you're feeling anxious about this procedure."

Therapeutic Communication Technique	Description	Examples
Focusing	Redirecting the patient to a key topic or concern	"Let's go back to what you mentioned about your pain level. Can you describe that more?"
Exploring	Delving deeper into a topic or emotion	"Tell me more about how you've been handling your stress."
Restating	Repeating back the patient's words to ensure clarity	"You said you feel unsure about the treatment. Is that right?"
Giving Recognition	Acknowledging the patient's efforts or achievements such as going through a treatment or decreasing blood pressure	"You've been really strong throughout this treatment process."

Example Case Review: Chronic Pain Patient

Scenario: Maria, a 59-year-old woman with chronic back pain, frequently requests opioid medications. During her monthly appointment, she becomes agitated when her request is denied and screams at the receptionist while checking in.

Possible Interventions and Discussion:
The NP can demonstrate empathy and understanding by beginning the conversation with, "I can see how much pain you're in, and I want to help you find relief." This approach validates Maria's pain and helps reduce her defensiveness. The NP can then collaborate with Maria to develop a comprehensive pain management plan that includes input from a multidisciplinary team, such as a pain specialist and physical therapist. Involving Maria in the planning process ensures that her concerns are addressed respectfully. Additionally, providing ongoing support through counseling or support groups can help address any challenges she may face.

Assignment: Therapeutic Communication
Goal: To apply patient-centered care principles and therapeutic communication strategies to effectively manage challenging patient interactions.

Objectives:

1. Apply therapeutic communication techniques to effectively de-escalate a tense patient interaction.
2. Demonstrate active listening skills during a patient interaction to validate the patient's concerns and emotions.

3. Analyze the situation to identify the underlying factors contributing to the patient's frustration.

Assignment Instructions: Read the case and answer the questions.

Case: A 45-year-old male patient Mr. Vessel arrives at the clinic for his scheduled follow-up appointment for uncontrolled hypertension. Upon entering the room, Mr. Vessel appears visibly agitated. He is raising his voice to others, expressing that his blood pressure has not improved despite taking his medication. He is frustrated and pacing the floor saying nobody is listening to him.

As the NP enters, Mr. Adams immediately starts venting his frustration, blaming the staff and medications for his lack of improvement. The NP is tasked with de-escalating the situation, addressing his concerns, and maintaining patient safety.

Discussion Questions:

1. What steps should the nurse practitioner take to initially de-escalate the patient's frustration? Hint: Use empathy in your talk. Give specific examples of what to say.
2. How can the nurse practitioner demonstrate therapeutic communication with the interaction with Mr. Adams? Use two examples for this question.
3. What strategies could the nurse practitioner employ to prevent the situation from escalating further while ensuring patient safety?
4. How might the NP analyze the factors contributing to Mr. Adams' frustration, and what could be included in the care plan moving forward?

(continued)

(continued)

Criteria	Excellent (10–9 Points)	Good (8–7 Points)	Fair (6–5 Points)	Needs Improvement or Not Done (4–0 Points)
De-escalation Techniques	Provides clear, effective de-escalation steps with specific, empathetic language examples.	Suggests appropriate de-escalation steps with some examples of empathetic language.	Lists basic de-escalation steps; lacking specificity in empathetic communication.	De-escalation steps are unclear, ineffective, lack empathy or nothing (zero).
Therapeutic Communication	Demonstrates strong understanding of therapeutic communication with two relevant examples.	Provides two examples of therapeutic communication, though may lack depth.	Gives basic examples of therapeutic communication, but lacks clarity or relevance.	Therapeutic communication examples are vague, irrelevant, or missing.

Escalation Prevention	Proposes well-thought-out strategies for preventing further escalation, prioritizing safety.	Offers strategies for preventing escalation, focusing on patient safety.	Suggests basic strategies, but lack focus on safety or detail.	Strategies for escalation prevention are unclear, ineffective, or missing.
Care Plan Analysis	Analyzes factors thoroughly and proposes a comprehensive, patient-centered care plan.	Analyzes factors and suggests a care plan, though may lack some detail or depth.	Provides a basic analysis and care plan, with limited patient-centered focus.	Analysis of factors is minimal, and the care plan is under-developed or unclear.
Clarity and Organization	Well-organized, clear, and concise answers that are easy to follow.	Generally well-organized and clear, with minor errors in organization or clarity.	Some organization, but answers may be unclear with missing elements.	Poorly organized, with unclear or missing answers

Total: 50 points.

6.3   Conclusion

The successful management of patient interactions, particularly in challenging scenarios, requires a holistic approach that combines clinical expertise with a deep understanding of psychological principles and effective communication strategies. Empathy is foundational in building trust and fostering strong patient–provider relationships. By employing strategies such as active listening, compassion, and motivational interviewing (MI), NPs can address patients' emotional and cognitive needs, ultimately leading to better adherence to treatment plans.

6.4   Professional Practice Guided by Evidence

By, Gina Myers PhD, RN

The importance of patient-centered care is at the core of NP practice and is closely intertwined with the use of evidence to guide clinical decisions. This was undoubtedly emphasized throughout the NP program. In fact, it is articulated at all levels of the AACNs Essentials of Professional Nursing Practice with evidence-based practice being defined as "a conscientious, problem-solving approach to clinical practice that incorporates the best evidence from well-designed studies, patient values and preferences, and a clinician's expertise in making decisions regarding a patient's care. Being knowledgeable about evidence-based practice and levels of evidence is important for clinicians to be confident about how much emphasis they should place on a study, report, practice alert or practice guideline when making decisions about a patient's care" [14]. This aligns with the knowledge and skills one received while in the NP program. When practicing at a higher level, using evidence in practice has never been more critical. As a provider, the NP will be the person registered nurses (RNs), colleagues, patients, and families look to for guidance on approaches to health; these same people may also challenge those decisions. Being confident in how to use research evidence to inform and support clinical decisions, while taking patient preference and personal clinical expertise into consideration, is crucial for success in this role.

6.4.1   Using Patient-Centered Evidence in Practice

While it is paramount to base practice approaches on evidence, it cannot always be done with tunnel vision. It is important to include the patient in a discussion of the treatment plan, explaining the best approach to care using research-based guidelines. The approach must be a balance of explaining and teaching, while allowing time for questions and listening to answers, observing for non-verbal cues that may reveal fear or confusion, and involving the patient in the prescribed regimen [15, 16]. Guideline recommendations are most successful when followed, so ensuring patients and families are willing and able to carry out the treatment plan is pivotal. When having discussions with patients, bring in questions related to their ability to engage in their own care, identifying any barriers that may exist related to physical, social, or cultural issues. Then, offer options in places where guidelines are flexible or alternatives exist.

For example, consider a cancer patient prone to blood clots who is having difficulty taking the prescribed Eliquis (apixaban) twice a day, reporting that it makes them feel unsteady in the morning. In response, the patient reduced the dosage to one dose at bedtime and asked if the full dose could be taken once a day instead of twice. The NP stresses that the recommended dosing is twice a day. However, the patient continues to express discomfort with the morning dose. An alternative, Xarelto (rivaroxaban) which can be taken once daily at night, is considered. This option is acceptable to the patient and still adheres to clinical guidelines for the treatment of cancer-related thrombosis [17].

6.4.2 Smooth Ways to Integrate Evidence

Being immersed in the required coursework for the NP program makes it somewhat easier to integrate evidence into practice due to mandatory assignments, time to investigate, and time to work on case studies. There is great benefit in working with a preceptor or having a lower patient load while accruing clinical hours. Once independent practice begins, the amount of time available to spend searching for research evidence decreases. This is especially true during the time as a novice NP, where one may encounter any number of "firsts" in a given day or week. To work most efficiently, the NP may want to invest in a clinically focused tool that provides practitioners with summary practice statements that are brief, easy to digest by being computer-based with an accompanying application for the phone or tablet. Some of the most popular tools are UpToDate and DynaMed. Recommendations found in clinically focused tools are based on clinical practice guidelines (CPG), systematic reviews (SR), and meta-analyses and often provide a robust reference list to support recommendations and for further reading [18].

6.4.3   Evidence Summaries and Clinical Practice Guidelines

Evidence summaries are an easy way to find large amounts of research evidence that have been appraised, analyzed, and summarized. This significantly reduces the effort to research a practice problem or answer a practice question. The first most useful piece of evidence to look for is a CPG. These can be found through a number of sources.

Sources

US Preventative Services Task Force
Cochrane Library
Johanna Briggs Institute
Guidelines UK
Centre for Evidence-based Medicine
JAMA evidence

CPGs provide summary statements based on SRs, meta-analyses, or large randomized controlled trials (RCT). A particularly helpful feature is that each recommendation is graded, allowing the NP to discern the amount of high-quality evidence to support it. Each organization uses a slightly different grading system and criteria, but all are similar in nature. The rating system is usually provided up front so the reader is easily able to understand the scores provided. While the evidence included in a CPG is appraised by the group creating the guideline, the reader will still need to decide the overall quality of the CPG provided. This is especially important if more than one CPG exists to answer a practice question. The gold standard in CPG appraisal is produced by the AGREE Trust Organization. The AGREE II is a 25-item appraisal tool that identifies the important aspects of a CPG to ensure the guideline development process is transparent, includes all the necessary evidence, and is presented free of bias [19].

6.4.4 Systemic Reviews

SRs are another type of high-level evidence summary that can help an NP consume a large amount of research information about a practice question without needing to search, read, and appraise many research studies. In an SR, a focused clinical question or PICOT (Population, Intervention, Compariosn, Outcome, Time) question is asked, the literature is searched, and the PICOT question is answered using research evidence. A PICOT question is a structured clinical question that stands for population, intervention, comparison, outcome, and time, which helps focus research efforts and guides the search for evidence. This is different from a regular review of the literature since an SR is typically conducted by a team of researchers using a systematic, exhaustive, and well-documented search strategy so others can replicate the approach. A PRISMA flow diagram is often included for transparency. The SR includes only studies deemed as high-quality research and pertinent to the PICOT question. Each included study is appraised independently by at least two team members and a quality score is decided upon. This strategy differs from a traditional narrative review in which the search strategy is neither systematic nor exhaustive. Narrative reviews are useful at providing an overview of a topic, but should not be considered as the sole guiding force for a practice change or way to address a clinical problem. At the conclusion of the SR, the authors will attempt to answer the PICOT question and give direction for practice [20].

6.4.5   Meta-Analysis: Synthesizing Quantitative Results

A meta-analysis is similar to an SR in that a number of studies are brought together for analysis, but the difference is that the quantitative results of those studies are synthesized using statistical methods. A meta-analysis is conducted with studies that have similar designs such as RCTs or quasi-experimental research and summarize the effect of an intervention. The summary statistic allows the combination of all studies results making it as though one large study was conducted. Results are typically provided graphically in a chart called a forest plot which shows data for individual studies along with the overall result [21]. While it may seem overwhelming to review forest plot results, there are a number of sources that can help interpret what they mean. One helpful source can be found at `https://s4be.cochrane.org/blog/2016/07/11/tutorial-read-forest-plot`. Once one learns how to do this, it becomes easy to find the numbers one is looking for to help answer the PICOT question.

6.4.6   Combining Systematic Reviews and Meta-Analyses

SRs and meta-analyses can be standalone or done in combination. An SR that includes a meta-analysis is a great find. The purpose of the SR remains the same: to answer a practice question based on a systematic search for all types of research evidence, but might also take research studies with similar designs and conduct a meta-analysis using those study results. Since not all studies in an SR have the same design, you may not see all the studies combined statistically. With this format, you will benefit from the appraisal and synthesis of the included studies but also have access to meta-analytic results of the appropriate studies. It is not unusual for the SR to include many studies, but only statistically synthesize a handful in the meta-analysis. When reading an SR that does not include a meta-analysis, you will typically see authors comment on why they did not quantitatively combine study results. Reasons usually include poor quality of studies, or studies with similar designs but different interventions, or varied measurement of outcomes. Refraining from combining results of a study is appropriate for these reasons [22].

6.4.7   *Digging Deeper on Complex Practice Approaches*

There are times when the NP's practice problem or question may not be easily answered by the high-level evidence summaries found. This can be due to a specific patient situation involving their unique circumstances, beliefs, or culture. In these cases, it may be helpful to review the reference list of the evidence summaries reviewed to see if there are individual pieces of evidence that might address the question. One can also enlist the help of a science librarian at a local college if still affiliated, or the medical librarian at the healthcare organization where practice takes place. Research databases are readily available with online platforms, and many libraries now have robust online accessibility that allows connecting with a librarian for help around the clock [18]. If those avenues are not available, one can search for free evidence in databases such as PubMed or collaborate with colleagues or your organization to access research materials. Professional organizations may also have resources such as specialty guidelines or databases as part of membership. In addition, a local NP Association may provide information on topics that are important. For example, the Nurse Practitioner Association of New York has a repository of past presentation abstracts, as well as educational topics that might be pertinent to addressing the practice issue. Professional connections and networking can also provide insight about available evidence. This is especially helpful if no research evidence is available to address a given problem.

6.5   Conclusion

Every NP strives to deliver exceptional patient-centered care. This care is best achieved through the integration of research evidence that is tailored to meet the individual patient's needs. The use of evidence summaries such as CPGs and SRs allows NPs to efficiently access and apply the best available evidence, even within the fast-paced environment of modern healthcare. By incorporating these tools into practice, NPs can support positive patient outcomes, ensuring that care is both scientifically grounded and responsive to patient needs.

6.6   Ethical Considerations

6.6.1   Introduction

Navigating the ethical challenges is essential in nursing practice, particularly for NPs who frequently encounter clinical and moral dilemmas. Ethical practice involves adhering to fundamental principles such as beneficence, non-maleficence, autonomy, and justice [23]. These principles guide NPs by prioritizing patient welfare while respecting patient autonomy and ensuring equity. Understanding and applying these principles in clinical settings helps NPs resolve ethical conflicts effectively and uphold professional integrity. An NP should always act in the patient's best interest, such as advocating for a second opinion, even if it involves challenging a colleague's decision. These core principles form the foundation for ethical decision-making in patient care.

6.6.2 Ethical Principles

In healthcare, several foundational ethical principles guide clinical decision-making and patient care, ensuring that NPs uphold their moral obligations while addressing complex medical situations. The principle of beneficence highlights a healthcare provider's obligation to not only prevent harm but also to actively promote the patient's well-being [23]. Non-maleficence requires providers to avoid causing harm and carefully weigh the risks and benefits of treatments. Autonomy underscores the importance of respecting patients' decision-making rights, necessitating informed consent, truth-telling, and confidentiality. Justice focuses on the fair distribution of healthcare resources, ensuring equitable treatment for all patients.

The following section discusses the application of these principles in practice, including strategies for resolving conflicts when ethical principles collide. Several illustrative cases will highlight common ethical dilemmas and their resolution, demonstrating the practical application of these moral principles.

Varkey (2021) provides examples of ethical conflicts and steps to resolve them [23].

Case 1:   Autonomy Vs. Beneficence

A 56-year-old male smoker with a solitary lung mass, suspected to be cancerous, declines a recommended biopsy and surgery despite being fully informed of the potential consequences.

Discussion

In addressing this conflict, the provider took several key steps to respect the patient's autonomy while upholding the principle of beneficence. First, the provider thoroughly explained the importance of the biopsy and surgery, as well as the risks associated with refusing treatment. Despite being fully informed and mentally competent, the patient declined the procedure due to a fear of surgery.

In this case, the principle of autonomy took precedence over beneficence. The provider respected the patient's decision. They ensured continued care by offering regular follow-up visits and monitoring. Additionally, the provider encouraged the patient to reconsider his decision and seek a second opinion, maintaining a supportive and proactive approach to managing the patient's healthcare while respecting his right to refuse treatment.

Case 2:   Non-maleficence Vs. Autonomy

A 20-year-old college student diagnosed with bacterial meningitis refuses treatment, despite being fully informed of the severe risk to his life.

Discussion

When non-maleficence (the obligation to prevent harm) conflicts with autonomy (the patient's right to make their own decisions), healthcare providers must proceed with caution. In this case, the provider first assessed the patient's mental capacity, considering the possibility of impaired judgment due to the seriousness of the illness.

Given the life-threatening risks and the concern that the patient's decision-making might be compromised, the provider chose to proceed with treatment despite the refusal, recognizing that the patient's refusal could be influenced by temporary mental incapacity. In this instance, the provider prioritized beneficence (saving the patient's life) over autonomy (the patient's choice). The provider continued to closely monitor and support the patient, ensuring that ethical care was maintained throughout the course of treatment.

Case 3:   Justice Vs. Beneficence

During a pandemic, two patients with severe respiratory failure both require the only available ventilator.

Discussion

In critical situations where medical resources are scarce, healthcare providers face difficult decisions that require balancing justice (the fair distribution of resources) with beneficence (acting in the patient's best interest). The allocation of the ventilator required an evaluation of which patient would benefit most, considering factors such as life expectancy, likelihood of survival, and potential future contributions.

In this case, the ventilator was ultimately allocated to the younger patient, who had a higher chance of survival and a longer life expectancy. The decision was guided by the principle of maximizing benefits—allocating the scarce resource to the patient with the best prospects for recovery—while also striving to ensure fairness. Though challenging, this approach aimed to achieve the greatest overall benefit within the constraints of limited medical resources.

Case 4:   Non-maleficence Vs. Beneficence

A 71-year-old man with end-stage COPD and multiple organ failure is on life support. Further treatment has been deemed futile.

Discussion

In end-of-life care, the ethical principles of non-maleficence (avoiding harm) and beneficence (acting in the patient's best interest) must be carefully balanced. In this case, the medical team faced the difficult decision of whether to continue life-sustaining treatment for a patient with a poor prognosis. The team thoroughly discussed the situation with the patient's family, ensuring they were fully informed about the futility of further aggressive treatment and the burdens versus benefits of life-sustaining interventions.

The decision was made to discontinue life support and transition to palliative care, prioritizing the patient's comfort and dignity in his remaining time. This resolution reflects a balance between non-maleficence, by avoiding further harm and unnecessary interventions, and beneficence, by focusing on providing compassionate care that promotes comfort at the end of life.

6.7   Conclusion

Resolving ethical conflicts in clinical practice is not just about applying principles; it's about understanding the deeper nuances of each situation. NPs must take the time to reflect on what truly matters for each patient, considering their unique circumstances, personal values, and the potential outcomes of different decisions. In these complex moments, reaching out to colleagues—whether ethicists, specialists, or social workers—can offer fresh insights and emotional support as you navigate difficult choices. Involving patients and their families in these discussions ensures that decisions are not only ethically sound but also compassionate and respectful of the individual's autonomy.

For NPs, facing these ethical challenges is an integral part of providing patient-centered care. By thoughtfully addressing these dilemmas, NPs become stronger advocates for their patients and remain aligned with the core values that shape their profession.

6.8   Patient Education for Nurse Practitioners

6.8.1   Introduction

Patient education is a critical component of the NP role, particularly for those in their first year of practice. Effective patient education can improve health outcomes, enhance patient satisfaction, and empower individuals to take control of their health [24]. For new NPs, understanding how to integrate patient education into clinical encounters is essential. This involves applying educational theories and frameworks to create meaningful and impactful learning experiences for patients.

6.8.2 NP Foundation

The role of the NP centers on health promotion and disease prevention, which are fundamental to nursing practice [25]. One of the key competencies expected of NPs upon graduation is the ability to educate patients. This includes assessing patients' educational needs, creating an effective learning environment, and coaching patients for behavior changes. The curriculum of NP preparation programs includes components such as pharmacology, assessment, and pathophysiology, all built on a strong foundation of health promotion for both ill and healthy patients. This foundation will be further strengthened in the future with Doctor of Nursing Practice (DNP) programs, which place special emphasis on health promotion [25].

Patient education involves informing, instructing, and guiding patients about their health conditions, treatment plans, and lifestyle modifications. It helps patients make informed decisions, adhere to treatments, and engage in preventive health behaviors. For first-year NPs, mastering patient education builds trust, promotes compliance, and empowers patients, leading to better health outcomes.

6.8.3 Theory

Theories can help explain how individuals learn in different settings. The optimal result of patient education is a change in behavior that stems not only from the transfer of knowledge but also from actively involving the patient in facilitating this change. Theories offer essential insights into how adults learn and how behavioral change can be encouraged, particularly in the context of patient education. Effective patient education goes beyond merely transferring knowledge; it requires actively engaging patients in the process to foster meaningful change [24]. This change is multifaceted and can be better understood through various models and theories that help explain motivation and patient behavior.

6.8.3.1   Health Belief Model

The Health Belief Model (HBM) is a framework used to explain and predict individual health behaviors by focusing on the attitudes and beliefs people have about health conditions [26]. The model suggests that a person's health behaviors are influenced by their perceived severity and susceptibility of a health issue, the benefits of acting, and barriers that might prevent them from taking that action [26]. Providers can effectively apply the HBM to guide patient education and encourage positive health behaviors.

This chart breaks down the HBM Components with examples:

Health Belief Model Component	Explanation	Example: Patient with Asthma
Severity	Discuss the seriousness of the health condition and its potential complications.	Explain the potential risks of uncontrolled asthma, such as severe asthma attacks or frequent hospital visits.

(continued)

Health Belief Model Component	Explanation	Example: Patient with Asthma
Susceptibility	Highlight the individual's risk factors and how they contribute to their condition.	Discuss how smoking or exposure to pollution can worsen the patient's asthma, increasing the likelihood of severe symptoms.
Benefits	Explain the positive outcomes of taking preventive or corrective action.	Emphasize how regular use of an inhaler can prevent asthma symptoms, reduce hospital visits, and improve overall quality of life.
Barriers	Identify and address obstacles that might prevent the patient from following the recommended action. Is there an issue with understanding the condition, cost of medication, side effects?	Address the patient's concerns about the cost of the inhaler and side effects. Offer solutions, such as generic inhalers if applicable or financial assistance programs.

Application of the Health Belief Model

The HBM serves as an effective framework for NPs to guide patients in understanding and managing their health [26]. For example, when working with a patient who has a diagnosis of hypertension, the NP can utilize the HBM by addressing each of its components. First, the NP can explain the severity of uncontrolled high blood pressure, discussing the increased risks of heart attack, stroke, and kidney disease. Next, the NP can discuss the patient's susceptibility of disease by emphasizing individual risk factors such as family history, diet, and physical inactivity. By personalizing the conversation, the NP helps the patient understand how specific lifestyle factors and genetics contribute to their risk. The NP would then highlight the benefits of managing blood pressure effectively, including medications, a healthy diet, and regular exercise can reduce complications and improve overall well-being. Finally, the NP would address any barriers to action, such as the patient's concerns about medication side effects or the difficulty of maintaining lifestyle changes. The NP can work with the patient to find tailored solutions, such as prescribing medications with fewer side effects, providing meal planning resources, or creating an exercise plan that fits the patient's schedule and preferences. By addressing these factors, the NP can help the patient feel more empowered and motivated to take control of their health.

6.8.3.2 Motivational Interviewing

Motivational Interviewing (MI) is an effective approach for discussing changes with patients, especially in clinical settings [27]. With extensive research exploring MI and its applications, this approach has gained widespread recognition for its effectiveness across various contexts. Unlike traditional methods of delivering information such as simply explaining the benefits of exercise, MI engages patients in a more interactive and collaborative conversation. Notably, MI can be conducted in as little as five minutes, making it a timely and efficient intervention for NPs to employ in clinical practice. By emphasizing respect for patient autonomy, compassion, and collaboration, MI allows NPs to guide patients through the stages of change, helping them resolve ambivalence and explore their own motivations for behavior change.

Core Skills of Motivational Interviewing

Motivational Interviewing (MI) relies on several core skills that foster patient engagement and positive change. These include asking open-ended questions, offering affirmations, reflective listening, and summarizing. Open-ended questions invite patients to share their thoughts and feelings, such as, "How do you feel about your current health?" or "What advantages do you see in quitting smoking?" [28]. Affirmations highlight the patient's strengths and past successes to build confidence. For example, the NP might say, "You were successful with losing weight in the past; tell me about that time." Reflective listening involves paraphrasing the patient's statements to demonstrate understanding, such as, "You're not sure about the diagnosis of PTSD" [28]. Summarizing helps consolidate discussions and reinforces key points, as in, "If I understand you correctly, you were successful in the past by walking every day, and you think you can get back on track by getting up early before work." Together, these skills create a supportive, collaborative environment that encourages patients to engage in meaningful behavior change [27].

The Four Processes of Motivational Interviewing

Motivational interviewing is structured around four processes: engaging, focusing, evoking, and planning [29]. Each process plays a crucial role in guiding the patient toward making positive changes. Engaging involves establishing a trusting, respectful, and therapeutic relationship where the patient feels welcomed and involved in mutual goal setting. Focusing helps maintain direction and aligns both the patient's and the provider's goals. Evoking is the process of encouraging "change talk," where the patient expresses their desire for change through statements like "I can," "I wish," or "I want." Finally, planning involves helping the patient develop a specific, measurable action plan that they are willing to implement. When patients resist discussing certain topics, such as diet, the NP can leave the door open for future conversations, ensuring the patient feels in control of their journey while keeping communication lines open [28]. Unlike traditional methods, which often involve a one-way transfer of information, motivational interviewing focuses on engaging patients in a conversation, making it both effective and efficient.

Example: An NP meets with John, a patient who is ambivalent about losing weight. The chart below breaks down the four processes of Motivational interviewing with examples for each:

Process	Description	Example	Provider Questions
Engaging	Establishing a trusting and respectful relationship.	The NP meets with John, a patient ambivalent about losing weight, and asks open-ended questions about his daily routine and health. This builds rapport and shows respect for John's perspective.	"Can you tell me about a typical day for you?" "How do you feel about your current health and lifestyle?"
Focusing	Setting an agenda that aligns with both patient and provider goals.	During a follow-up visit, John expresses his desire to improve his diet. The NP and John agree to focus their discussions on dietary changes and set specific goals.	"What are some goals you'd like to focus on for the next few months?" "How would you feel about making changes to your diet?"

Process	Description	Example	Provider Questions
Evoking	Eliciting the patient's motivations for change through "change talk."	The NP asks John, "What are some reasons you want to improve your diet?" John responds, "I want to feel better and have more energy." The NP affirms this motivation and encourages John to express more.	"What benefits do you think you'll experience by improving your diet?" "What motivates you to make this change now?"
Planning	Developing a specific and measurable action plan that the patient is willing to implement.	The NP and John work together to create a realistic plan for dietary change. Replacing sugary snacks with fruits. Schedule weekly check-ins to monitor progress and show support.	"What small changes do you feel confident about starting with?" "How can we track your progress in a way that works for you?"

Role-Play Exercise

Purpose: The purpose of this exercise is to help NPs practice and refine their motivational interviewing skills, particularly in addressing patient ambivalence. By engaging in this role-play, participants will learn how to guide patients through the process of identifying and resolving their conflicting feelings, ultimately empowering them to make positive health changes.

Case: Consider a patient, Kadia, who wants to lose weight but loves bacon and hates exercising. Kadia exhibits ambivalence—wanting to change yet reluctant to give up certain habits. An NP can use motivational interviewing to explore Kadia's feelings and motivations, helping her resolve this ambivalence.

Engage in a Collaborative Conversation: Start by building a trusting relationship with Kadia, creating a safe space where she feels comfortable discussing her concerns.

Identify Kadia's Goals and Motivations: Use open-ended questions to gain insight into Kadia's perspective, understanding what drives her desire to lose weight and what challenges she faces.

Elicit Change Talk: Encourage Kadia to articulate her reasons for wanting to lose weight, focusing on the positive outcomes she hopes to achieve.

Develop a Specific Action Plan: Collaborate with Kadia to create a realistic and measurable plan that aligns with her goals, ensuring that it is both achievable and sustainable.

6.8.3.3 Keller's Motivational Theory

Keller's Motivational Theory is another approach that involves the learner. It emphasizes four key components to effectively engage and motivate individuals: attention, relevance, confidence, and satisfaction [30]. Attention captures and maintains a person's interest, often achieved by using a variety of teaching methods. If a learner loses focus, their motivation to act may diminish. Relevance connects new knowledge to the patient's existing life experiences, making it easier for them to understand and apply the information. By learning more about the patient's life, healthcare providers can personalize education, which fosters greater confidence and satisfaction. Building confidence through the use of smaller milestones toward a larger goal helps patients feel a sense of achievement. Providing praise reinforces this confidence. Finally, satisfaction, whether intrinsic or extrinsic, plays a vital role in sustaining motivation, encouraging patients to stay engaged and committed to their health goals.

Application to Practice

Keller's Motivational Theory can be effectively applied in various healthcare settings to enhance patient education and motivation. For example, in a psychiatric practice, an NP can use this theory to educate and motivate patients by focusing on the four key components: attention, relevance, confidence, and satisfaction. Consider a patient diagnosed with depression who is struggling to adhere to an exercise regimen that could improve their mood. The NP can apply Keller's theory in the following ways:

Attention: The NP begins with an open, empathetic conversation about the patient's feelings and daily activities, using tools like visuals or apps to keep the discussion engaging and to demonstrate how exercise can positively impact their mental health.

Relevance: The NP personalizes the information by connecting the benefits of exercise to the patient's own life. For instance, the NP might remind the patient of times when they felt better after being active and suggest enjoyable activities like walking the dog or gardening. The NP could ask, "Tell me about a time when you felt good and were more active," to focus on positive experiences to build upon.

Confidence: Rather than overwhelming the patient with large goals, the NP breaks the plan into manageable steps, such as starting with a 10-minute walk each day. Celebrating these small wins reinforces the patient's belief that progress is achievable, building their confidence.

Satisfaction: To sustain motivation, the NP offers praise and encouragement throughout the process, emphasizing both the immediate rewards (feeling slightly better) and the long-term benefits (positive feedback from loved ones or reduced anxiety).

By following Keller's approach, the NP can make the education process more effective, helping the patient feel motivated and engaged in their own care.

6.9   Conclusion

Patient education is a cornerstone of NP practice, particularly in the early years when establishing a foundation in health promotion and disease prevention. As new NPs integrate patient education into clinical encounters, they can draw upon established frameworks like the HBM and motivational theories to facilitate meaningful behavioral change. By applying these frameworks, NPs can tailor their approach to meet the unique needs of each patient, enhancing both understanding and engagement.

Motivational interviewing (MI) stands out as a highly effective, patient-centered approach that enables NPs to navigate complex health behaviors while respecting the patient's autonomy. Unlike traditional, directive methods, MI fosters a collaborative dialogue that empowers patients to explore their motivations and take ownership of their health decisions. As NPs gain experience and reflect on their practice, they can continue to refine their patient education techniques, making them more adaptive and responsive to individual patient needs.

Ultimately, patient education is not just about conveying information—it's about building trust, fostering empowerment, and supporting patients in making informed decisions that improve their overall well-being. Through thoughtful use of evidence-based frameworks and techniques, NPs can make a lasting impact on their patients' health outcomes.

6.10 Diversity, Equity, and Inclusion

DEI refers to the efforts and strategies focused on fostering an environment that values difference, promotes fairness, and cultivates a sense of belonging for all individuals [31]. Diversity acknowledges the presence of various characteristics and identities such as race, ethnicity, gender, sexual orientation, age, disability, and socioeconomic background, as well as recognizing multiple perspectives. Equity focuses on ensuring fair treatment, opportunities, and access for all people. This is accomplished by addressing systemic inequalities and removing barriers to participation. Inclusion creates an atmosphere where every individual feels respected and welcomed. It empowers one to contribute fully, ensuring that diversity is effectively supported within an organization. DEI initiatives are critical to promoting justice and enhancing the quality of care in healthcare and other professional environments [31].

6.10.1   Cultural Competence

Cultural competence supports the entire DEI effort, as it assists individuals with the tools to implement these principles. Cultural competence refers to the ability to effectively integrate knowledge, attitudes, and policies that value diversity of the people they serve [32]. It is a process that involves transforming knowledge about different groups of people into standards and practices. This strives to improve the quality and healthcare outcomes of all [32]. Without cultural competence, diversity efforts can fall short, equity may be compromised, and inclusion may lack depth. Providing culturally competent care means being respectful of and responsive to the cultural and linguistic needs of patients. Acknowledging and respecting diverse cultural backgrounds ensures that care is delivered in a culturally sensitive manner [33].

The foundation of cultural competence is care that is patient-centered. It starts with developing a rapport with clear communication while assessing the characteristics of the patient as well as their beliefs and background [33]. Building this relationship involves therapeutic techniques such as active listening and open communication. These techniques contribute to understanding and addressing the concerns of patients who may be hesitant to certain aspects of their care.

Despite the progress in cultural competence, significant gaps remain, particularly in specialties like internal medicine, pediatrics, and critical care. Training programs often lack effective curricula to address the care of patients with limited English proficiency (LEP) or from underrepresented groups. While diversity plans exist, racial and ethnic diversity among trainees and faculty remains limited. Furthermore, the critical care workforce has seen persistently low numbers of women and minorities, underscoring the need for more targeted interventions to address these disparities [34].

6.10.2 DEI and Outcomes

DEI initiatives in healthcare contribute significantly to improved patient outcomes by fostering an environment that is culturally sensitive, reduces health disparities, and ensures that care is patient centered. Studies indicate that healthcare teams with diverse members are better equipped to understand and address the unique needs of various patient populations, leading to improved communication, greater patient satisfaction, and better adherence to treatment plans. Equity efforts help reduce barriers to care, ensuring all patients, regardless of background, have access to high-quality care, which is linked to better outcomes, especially in marginalized groups [35]. Additionally, inclusive practices in healthcare settings promote trust and respect between patients and providers, which is crucial for effective care.

6.10.2.1   Application to the NP

To effectively apply these DEI principles, NPs play a critical
role in bridging gaps in communication and cultural understanding, ensuring that all patients receive equitable and
respectful care. For example, the NP may encounter patients
who speak limited English, which can create significant
challenges in ensuring they understand their diagnosis and
treatment plan, potentially leading to non-compliance. In
such cases, using a professional interpreter is essential for
facilitating accurate communication between the provider
and the patient. Interpreters can be utilized in person or via
phone, ensuring that language barriers do not compromise
the quality of care provided. Respecting the patient's language and cultural background is crucial, as it fosters trust
and helps improve health outcomes [36]. Additionally, there
are legal obligations that healthcare providers must adhere
to regarding interpreter services. US federal laws, such as the
Americans with Disabilities Act (ADA) and Title VI of the
Civil Rights Act of 1964, require healthcare providers to offer
appropriate auxiliary aids and services, including qualified
interpreters, to ensure effective communication with patients
who have LEP or are deaf or hard of hearing [36]. Compliance with these laws not only fulfills legal requirements but
also upholds the principles of patient-centered care. When
language barriers exist, patients still want their providers to
make an effort to communicate and demonstrate kindness
and respect. Simple steps such as training providers in empathy and improving communication strategies such as this
helps ensure patients feel respected and acknowledged [37].

NPs play a significant role in delivering care to patients
from diverse backgrounds, including race, ethnicity, gender,

sexual orientation, or socioeconomic status. Diversity in healthcare also includes factors such as age, with patients ranging from infants to the elderly, each presenting unique health needs and communication styles. NPs must also consider patients with disabilities—whether physical, cognitive, or sensory—who require accessible communication and tailored care. Language and literacy differences further complicate care, often necessitating the use of interpreters or simplified medical explanations [24]. Additionally, NPs encounter patients with neurological or psychological differences, such as autism, ADHD, depression, or anxiety, who may need extra time, patience, and support to feel at ease. By recognizing and adapting to these varied needs, NPs foster trust, strengthen relationships, and support better health outcomes.

Equity in healthcare means ensuring that all patients, regardless of their background, receive high-quality care [31]. NPs are uniquely positioned to address health disparities by identifying and overcoming barriers such as socioeconomic status, language differences, and geographic location. By providing equitable care, they help close gaps in health outcomes, ensuring that vulnerable populations receive the necessary services and interventions. Furthermore, inclusion is central to patient-centered care. NPs must create environments where every patient feels welcomed, respected, and heard. By practicing active listening, avoiding assumptions, and empowering patients to engage in their care decisions, NPs enhance communication, foster stronger relationships, and improve adherence to treatment plans, ultimately leading to better patient outcomes.

6.10.3   DEI Strategies

To ensure DEI is addressed, there are several strategies, including integrating DEI into the mission and vision of healthcare institutions and increasing regulatory requirements related to DEI as well as diversity in leadership [38]. Additionally, providing funding and mentoring programs to support providers from diverse backgrounds is essential to fostering diversity in leadership roles within the profession.

6.10.3.1   Workforce Diversity

The importance of integrating DEI into healthcare extends to the NP workforce itself. Over 75% of NPs and nurse midwives are White (Non-Hispanic), making them the most common racial group within the profession [38]. In contrast, Black (non-Hispanic) individuals represent only 8.72% of the NP workforce. This lack of diversity presents challenges in delivering culturally responsive care, particularly for patients from underrepresented communities who may feel alienated or mistrustful of the healthcare system due to past experiences of discrimination or bias. The underrepresentation of minority groups in the NP workforce perpetuates disparities in care quality, patient safety, and access to services [38].

Increasing diversity within the NP workforce is crucial for improving patient outcomes [38]. Advanced practice registered nurses (APRNs) from diverse backgrounds are more likely to work in underserved communities and contribute valuable perspectives to patient care, enhancing the cultural responsiveness of healthcare. However, the limited representation of APRNs of color in the workforce, particularly in faculty roles, continues to contribute to ongoing disparities in health outcomes and hinders the creation of a more inclusive healthcare environment.

6.10.3.2   Leadership, Mentoring, and Collaboration

Increasing diverse representation in leadership roles and improving data collection on the contributions and impact of APRNs of color are critical steps toward creating a more equitable and inclusive healthcare workforce [34]. By ensuring that the diversity of our communities is reflected in healthcare leadership and decision-making, we promote a more just and effective system. This approach emphasizes the need for diverse leadership at every level, integrating the values of inclusion into both strategic decisions and daily operations.

Best practices for advancing diversity in leadership have been outlined by various researchers. For example, Stanford (2020) highlighted the importance of ongoing learning, leveraging diversity for innovation, and aligning inclusion with organizational priorities [34].

NPs have a unique role in advocating for diversity and inclusion. For example, they can help champion policies that promote diversity and seek funding to eliminate barriers for marginalized communities. NPs can drive meaningful change. Additionally, they can start or support initiatives such as mentorship programs to help APRNs from underrepresented backgrounds enter and succeed in the profession. For example, mentorship programs like the Diversity in Nurse Anesthesia Mentorship Program (DNAMP) and the National Black Nurse Practitioner Association (NBNPA) play a crucial role in empowering APRNs from marginalized communities. The DNAMP, for instance, has grown to over 1,300 members, including CRNAs, SRNAs, RNs, and nursing students [39]. It focuses on supporting individuals from marginalized populations and preparing them for successful careers. Similarly, the NBNPA is dedicated to advancing NPs and addressing healthcare disparities in underserved communities through social fellowship and philanthropic efforts [40].

Promoting collaboration, shared goals, and mutual understanding among diverse communities is key to advancing DEI in healthcare. Other key strategies include organizing joint events, conferences, and community outreach programs that address health disparities. These initiatives bring together members of different professional organizations, allowing them to unite around shared missions, such as reducing healthcare inequities. By encouraging interprofessional collaboration through these events, NPs, and other healthcare professionals discuss best practices for patient care, cultural competence, and DEI issues. This helps break down silos and fosters unified efforts toward equity.

Transparency and Accountability

Transparency is key to sustaining DEI efforts. Organizations must openly report on DEI metrics and demonstrate the concrete steps they are taking to support DEI. Achieving equity requires a long-term commitment, continuing education, and a firm resolve to break down systemic barriers, making DEI a core part of company culture and daily operations [41]. Moving beyond diversity and inclusion efforts, the focus should be on achieving true equity—measurable and meaningful outcomes that address systemic racism and inequality [41].

To truly advance DEI, organizations need to embed it as a fundamental part of their overall strategy. Equity should be incorporated into performance metrics across departments, such as marketing, procurement, finance, and technology. Leadership plays a significant role in this process. Leaders must take ownership of DEI progress by setting clear goals, holding teams accountable, and consistently tracking outcomes such as workforce diversity and pay equity.

Accreditation Standards and Progress

Accreditation standards play a significant role in promoting DEI progress by setting clear expectations and fostering accountability within healthcare organizations. For example, the Liaison Committee on Medical Education (LCME) implemented diversity accreditation standards between 2012 and 2017, which contributed to an increase in female, Black, and Hispanic medical school matriculants in the United States [34]. However, sustained progress requires embedding diversity and inclusion principles into the core mission of healthcare organizations. Rather than simply appointing diversity officers, organizations must ensure these principles are woven into every aspect of their culture, where they are consistently measured, valued, and promoted. This approach involves engaging stakeholders at all levels, sharing successes and lessons learned with other organizations, and creating early exposure programs for underrepresented groups in local communities. By implementing these strategies, healthcare organizations can improve patient care outcomes and create better work environments for healthcare professionals [34].

6.10.3.3   Addressing Bias

Understanding and addressing unconscious bias is essential for healthcare providers, particularly new NPs as it plays a significant role in delivering equitable, patient-centered care. Unconscious, or implicit, bias refers to the automatic and often involuntary attitudes or stereotypes that influence our actions and decisions without our awareness [42]. These biases stem from the brain's natural tendency to categorize information quickly, relying on past experiences and cultural norms to make judgments [42]. In healthcare, such biases can subtly affect clinical decisions and patient interactions, potentially leading to disparities in care. For example, unconscious biases might influence how a diagnosis is made, which treatment options are offered, and how patients are communicated with and treated during their visits [43].

For new NPs, recognizing and mitigating these biases is crucial to providing high-quality, equitable care. When left unaddressed, unconscious biases can contribute to disparities in treatment, erode trust, and diminish the overall quality of care. Marginalized patients, for instance, might receive different treatment recommendations based on bias rather than clinical evidence, resulting in poorer health outcomes [44]. Additionally, when patients perceive bias or unfair treatment, they may lose trust in the healthcare system, leading to lower adherence to treatment plans and reduced engagement in follow-up care [45].

Self-Awareness and Reflection

Cultivating self-awareness and engaging in continuous education are key strategies for healthcare providers to recognize and reduce unconscious bias, ultimately leading to more equitable patient care. The journey to addressing unconscious bias begins with self-awareness. Regular reflection on one's thoughts, attitudes, and behaviors are crucial for identifying potential biases [46]. Tools like the Implicit Association Test (IAT) can be particularly helpful in uncovering hidden biases by measuring the strength of associations between different concepts [47]. Additionally, practices such as reflective journaling and mindfulness can enhance a provider's awareness of automatic reactions and judgments during patient interactions, paving the way for more objective and equitable care [48].

Education and Training

Ongoing education and training in diversity, equity, inclusion (DEI), and cultural competency are essential for mitigating unconscious bias. Cultural competency training equips healthcare providers with strategies to manage biases and deliver more effective care to diverse populations. This training not only raises awareness of personal biases but also provides practical tools for improving communication, patient engagement, and clinical decision-making. In recognition of its importance, some US states, including California and New Jersey, now mandate cultural competency training for healthcare professionals as part of their licensure requirements. These mandates highlight the growing emphasis on improving patient care quality through such education, ensuring that healthcare providers are better prepared to serve diverse communities [49].

Assignment: Harvard Implicit Bias Test and Reflection

Goal: This assignment is designed to encourage critical self-reflection and practical application of the insights gained from the test to the role as an NP.

(continued)

(continued)

Objectives

1. **Analyze** your own unconscious biases by engaging with the Harvard Implicit Association Test (IAT) and reflecting on the results.
2. **Develop** strategies to minimize the impact of unconscious biases in your clinical practice as an NP.

Instructions:

1. **Choose a Test:**
   Visit the Harvard Implicit Bias Test website at https://implicit.harvard.edu/implicit and select one IAT that interests you (e.g., Gender, Race, Age, Religion, etc.).
2. **Complete the Test:**
   Follow the instructions to complete the selected Implicit Association Test.
3. **Reflect:**
   After completing the test, answer the following reflection questions in a 2-page paper:

Reflection Questions:

4. What were your initial thoughts before taking the test, and how did you feel about the topic you chose?
5. What were the results of your test, and did they align with your expectations? Why or why not?
6. How might the awareness of your unconscious biases influence your interactions with patients? What strategies can you implement to minimize the impact of these biases in your practice?

Rubric

Criteria	Excellent (10 pts)	Good (8 pts)	Fair (6 pts)	Needs Improvement (4 pts)
Test Completion	Completed the IAT thoroughly and thoughtfully chose a test that challenges assumptions.	Completed the IAT with moderate reflection on the test choice.	Completed the IAT but with limited reflection on the test choice.	Incomplete or superficial engagement with the IAT.
Reflection Depth	Provided deep insights into biases, with clear connections to NP practice.	Reflected on biases with some connection to NP practice.	Reflection lacks depth or connection to NP practice.	Minimal reflection with no connection to NP practice.
Writing Quality	Well-organized, clear, and free of errors.	Organized with minor errors.	Some organization issues and several errors.	Poorly organized with significant errors.

6.11   Conclusion

Patient-centered care is the cornerstone of effective NP practice, requiring a blend of empathy, cultural competence, therapeutic communication, and ethical decision-making. Equally important is the integration of evidence-based practice, which supports the NP's ability to make informed clinical decisions. This chapter has explored various facets of patient-centered care, including the psychological principles that influence patient behavior and the significance of DEI in creating a welcoming environment for all patients. As healthcare continues to evolve in 2024, embracing DEI principles will not only enhance NP practice but also contribute to a more equitable and inclusive healthcare system. As NPs continue to develop their skills, integrating these elements into daily practice will enhance patient outcomes and foster stronger, more trusting relationships. By remaining committed to continuous learning, self-reflection, and collaboration, NPs will be well-equipped to navigate the complexities of patient care and make meaningful contributions to the ever-evolving healthcare landscape.

References

1. Epstein, R.M. and Street, R.L. Jr. (2011). The values and value of patient-centered care. *Ann. Fam. Med.* 9 (2): 100–103.
2. Street, R.L. Jr., Gordon, H.S., Ward, M.M. et al. (2009). Patient participation in medical consultations: why some patients are more involved than others. *Med. Care* 43 (10): 960–969.
3. Derksen, F., Bensing, J., and Lagro-Janssen, A. (2017). Effectiveness of empathy in general practice: a systematic review. *Br. J. Gen. Pract.* 63 (606): e76–e84.

4. Hong, Y.R. and Oh, H. (2019). The effects of patient-centered communication: exploring the mediating role of trust in healthcare quality among U.S. adults. *J Patient Exp.* 6 (3): 209–216.

5. Bertakis, K.D. and Azari, R. (2011). Patient-centered care is associated with decreased health care utilization. *J. Am. Board Fam. Med.* 24 (3): 229–239.

6. Turner, R.A. and Archer, L. (2020). How empathy and listening skills reduce anxiety in public healthcare settings. *J. Health Commun.* 25 (6): 565–573.

7. Bandura, A. (1997). *Self-Efficacy: The Exercise of Control.* New York: Freeman.

8. Li, S., Liu, X., Zheng, Z., and Liu, L. (2024). The role of self-efficacy in the relationship between body image and sleep quality among breast cancer patients. *Psychooncology* 33 (2): 223–232.

9. William, L. and Bond, M.J. (2002). Social support, self-efficacy, and adherence to diabetes self-care: a study of minority adults. *Diabetes Care* 25 (10): 1736–1741.

10. Stein, D., Cannity, K., Weiner, R. et al. (2022). General and unique communication skills challenges for advanced practice providers: a mixed-methods study. *J. Adv. Pract. Oncol.* 13 (1): 32–43.

11. Dean, E. (2023). The de-escalation skills you need to handle conflict situations. *RCNi Journals* Available from: https://journals.rcni.com/mental-health-practice/evidence/the-deescalation-skills-you-need-to-handle-conflict-situations-mhp.26.6.19.s7 (accessed 30 August 2024).

12. Joint Commission (2019). Quick safety issue 47: de-escalation in health care. *The Joint Commission* Available from: https://www.jointcommission.org/resources/news-and-multimedia/newsletters/newsletters/quick-safety/quick-safety-issue-47-de-escalation-in-health-care (accessed 30 August 2024).

13. Doyle, C., Lennox, L., and Bell, D. (2013). A systematic review of evidence on the links between patient experience and clinical safety and effectiveness. *BMJ Open* 3 (1): e001570.

14. American Association of Colleges of Nursing (2021). *The Essentials: core Competencies for Professional Nursing Education.*

Washington, D.C.: AACN Available from: https://www. aacnnursing.org/Portals/0/PDFs/Publications/ Essentials-2021.pdf (accessed 5 September 2024).

15. Kvarnström, K., Westerholm, A., Airaksinen, M., and Liira, H. (2021). Factors contributing to medication adherence in patients with a chronic condition: a scoping review of qualitative research. *Pharmaceutics.* 13 (7): 1100. https://doi.org/10.3390/ pharmaceutics13071100.

16. Świątoniowska-Lonc, N., Polański, J., Tański, W., and Jankowska-Polańska, B. (2020). Impact of satisfaction with physician-patient communication on self-care and adherence in patients with hypertension: Cross-sectional study. *BMC Health Serv. Res.* 20 (1): 1046. https://doi.org/10.1186/s12913-020-05912-0.

17. Lyman, G.H., Carrier, M., Ay, C. et al. (2021). American Society of Hematology 2021 guidelines for management of venous thromboembolism: prevention and treatment in patients with cancer. *Blood Adv.* 5 (4): 927–974. https://doi.org/10.1182/ bloodadvances.2020003431.

18. Myers, G. and Young, V. (2025). The EBPI+ model search for evidence: mapping the journey. In: *The Evidence-Based Practice Improvement Model+: A Practical Guide for Success* (ed. R.F. Levin and B. Lauder). New York: Springer Publishing Company.

19. AGREE Trust (2024). Welcome to the AGREE enterprise website. AGREE Trust. https://www.agreetrust.org (accessed 5 September 2024).

20. Randles, R. and Finnegan, A. (2023). Guidelines for writing a systematic review. *Nurse Educ. Today* 125: 1–6. https://doi. org/10.1016/j.nedt.2023.105803.

21. Myung, S.K. (2023). How to review and assess a systematic review and meta-analysis article. *Sci Ed.* 10 (2): 119–126.

22. Lensen, S. (2023). When to pool data in a meta-analysis (and when not to)? *Fertil. Steril.* 119 (6): 902–903. https://doi. org/10.1016/j.fertnstert.2023.03.015.

23. Varkey, B. (2021). Principles of clinical ethics and their application to practice. *Med. Princ. Pract.* 30 (1): 17–28.

24. Bastable, S.B. (2023). *Nurse as Educator: Principles of Teaching and Learning for Nursing Practice*, 6e. Jones & Bartlett Learning.

25. Burman, M.E., Hart, A.M., Conley, V. et al. (2009). Reconceptualizing the core of nurse practitioner education and practice. *J. Am. Acad. Nurse Pract.* 21 (1): 11–17.
26. Glanz, K., Rimer, B.K., and Viswanath, K. (2015). *Health Behavior: Theory, Research, and Practice*, 5e. Jossey-Bass.
27. Koh-Knox, C.P. (2009). Motivational interviewing in health care: helping patients change behavior. *Am. J. Pharm. Educ.* 73 (7): 127.
28. Rollnick, S., Miller, W.R., and Butler, C.C. (2008). *Motivational Interviewing in Health Care: Helping Patients Change Behavior.* Guilford Press.
29. Miller, W.R. and Rollnick, S. (2013). *Motivational Interviewing: Helping People Change*, 3e. Guilford Press.
30. Keller, J.M. (1987). Development and use of the ARCS model of instructional design. *J. Instr. Dev.* 10 (3): 2–10.
31. National Institutes of Health (2021). *Diversity, Equity, and Inclusion Strategic Plan.* National Institutes of Health.
32. Centers for Disease Control and Prevention (2023). *Cultural Competence in Healthcare.* Centers for Disease Control and Prevention.
33. Biswas-Diener, R. and Diener, E. (2006). The subjective well-being of the homeless, and lessons for happiness. *Soc. Indic. Res.* 76 (2): 185–205.
34. Stanford, F.C. (2020). Diversity, equity, and inclusion in healthcare: lessons from a national survey. *J. Healthc. Manag.* 65 (5): 312–324.
35. Gomez, L.E. and Bernet, P. (2019). Diversity improves performance and outcomes. *J. Natl. Med. Assoc.* 111 (4): 383–392.
36. U.S. Department of Justice (2020). Americans with Disabilities Act and Title VI of the Civil Rights Act of 1964: effective communication. https://www.ada.gov/effective-comm.htm (accessed 30 August 2024).
37. Turner, R.E. and Archer, E. (2020). Patient-centered care: the patients' perspective—a mixed-methods pilot study. *Afr J Prim Health Care Fam Med.* 12 (1): e1–e8.
38. Carthon, J.M.B. (2022). Increasing diversity in the nursing workforce: a call to action. *J Nurs Regul.* 13 (3): 18–24.

39. Diversity in Nurse Anesthesia Mentorship Program (2024). Annual report: progress and impact. Diversity in Nurse Anesthesia Mentorship Program.

40. National Black Nurse Practitioner Association (2024). About us. https://nbnpa.enpnetwork.com/page/28021-about-us (accessed 30 August 2024).

41. Deloitte (2021). The equity imperative: the role of DEI in achieving measurable and meaningful outcomes. Deloitte.

42. FitzGerald, C. and Hurst, S. (2017). Implicit bias in healthcare professionals: a systematic review. *BMC Med Ethics.* 18 (1): 19.

43. Chapman, E.N., Kaatz, A., and Carnes, M. (2013). Physicians and implicit bias: how doctors may unwittingly perpetuate health care disparities. *J. Gen. Intern. Med.* 28 (11): 1504–1510.

44. Hall, W.J., Chapman, M.V., Lee, K.M. et al. (2015). Implicit racial/ ethnic bias among health care professionals and its influence on health care outcomes: a systematic review. *Am. J. Public Health* 105 (12): e60–e66.

45. Penner, L.A., Dovidio, J.F., West, T.V. et al. (2010). Aversive racism and medical interactions with black patients: a field study. *J. Exp. Soc. Psychol.* 46 (2): 436–440. https://doi.org/10.1016/ j.jesp.2009.11.004.

46. Carnes, M., Devine, P.G., Baier Manwell, L. et al. (2015). The effect of an intervention to break the gender bias habit for faculty at one institution: a cluster randomized, controlled trial. *Acad. Med.* 90 (2): 221–230.

47. Greenwald, A.G., McGhee, D.E., and Schwartz, J.L. (1998). Measuring individual differences in implicit cognition: the implicit association test. *J. Pers. Soc. Psychol.* 74 (6): 1464–1480.

48. Stone, J. and Moskowitz, G.B. (2011). Non-conscious bias in medical decision-making: what can be done to reduce it? *Med. Educ.* 45 (8): 768–776.

49. Betancourt, J.R., Green, A.R., Carrillo, J.E., and Ananeh-Firempong, O. (2016). Defining cultural competence: a practical framework for addressing racial/ethnic disparities in health and healthcare. *Public Health Rep.* 118 (4): 293–302.

Chapter 7
Self-Care

Mary Handley, PhD, LMHC, CRC
Le Moyne College Clinical Mental Health Counseling
Syracuse, NY, USA

Strength in the Storm: A Personal NP Story
Alyssa Sonneborn, FNP-BC
Le Moyne College, Syracuse NY, USA

Chapter Highlights

Self-Care
Burnout
Compassion Fatigue
Resilience
Emotional Intelligence

Nurse Practitioner: Transition Guide, First Edition. Sara L. Gleasman-DeSimone.
© 2025 John Wiley & Sons, Inc. Published 2025 by John Wiley & Sons, Inc.

7.1   Introduction

Caring for others in healthcare requires empathy, compassion, understanding, and unwavering commitment. Nurse practitioners (NPs) embody these qualities, which often draw them to the profession, leading them to devote much of their time to supporting others. To maintain their well-being in this demanding role, it is important to also prioritize self-care. This chapter not only highlights the importance of self-care but also delves into the challenges of burnout and compassion fatigue. It offers concrete strategies and resources to support NPs in sustaining mental health and resilience.

Objectives with Mapping to 2021 American Association of Colleges of Nursing (AACN) Masters Essentials

1. Analyze self-care and how it affects a work/life balance.
2. Domain 9: Personal, Professional, and Leadership Development.
3. Identify realistic strategies and resources for caring for oneself.
4. Domain 7: Interprofessional Partnerships.
5. Evaluate how burnout and compassion fatigue affect one's professional and personal life.
6. Domain 1: Knowledge for Nursing Practice.
7. Implement strategies for improved self-care at the workplace.
8. Domain 9: Personal, Professional, and Leadership Development.

"Self-care is giving the world the best of you, instead of what's left of you."—Katie Reed

7.2   Self-Care

Self-care involves intentional, deliberate actions aimed at nurturing one's mental, physical, or spiritual well-being [1]. Self-care has become a widely discussed topic in both the media and professional circles, with growing recognition of its importance in promoting a healthy work–life balance. Many professionals understand its significance, yet they often fail to implement it effectively or only practice it in the short term. In the healthcare field, particularly in nursing, consistent and purposeful self-care is crucial for maintaining job satisfaction, competence, and effectiveness. The American Nurses Association (ANA) Code of Ethics even outlines self-care as an ethical responsibility for nurses [2].

For NPs, self-care is essential to provide the high-quality care that patients need and deserve. Without it, NPs risk becoming overwhelmed, exhausted, and susceptible to burnout and compassion fatigue. This can severely hinder their ability to offer appropriate care to others [1]. To support their well-being and effectiveness, it is beneficial for NPs to regularly evaluate their own mental and physical health needs. One way an individual can assess this is through a self-care assessment tool. This allows NPs to identify their strengths and areas needing attention, forming the foundation of a realistic self-care plan. This plan can help NPs add intentional activities into their routine, better understand their personal needs, and improve their work–life balance.

7.2.1 Self-Care Assessment

A self-care assessment allows NPs to evaluate their current practices and identify areas that may require additional attention. The following worksheet for assessing self-care is not exhaustive, but rather suggestive [3]. Individuals are encouraged to add areas of self-care that are relevant to their personal needs and rate themselves on how often and how well they are tending to their well-being [3]. Upon completion, patterns in the responses should be observed. Are some areas of self-care receiving more attention, while others are being overlooked? Are there items on the list that had not previously been considered? It is important to listen to internal responses and reflections about self-care, taking note of any areas that may need to be prioritized moving forward.

Rate the Following Areas According to How Well You Think You Are Doing

3 = I do this well (e.g., frequently)
2 = I do this OK (e.g., occasionally)
1 = I barely or rarely do this
0 = I never do this
? = This never occurred to me

Physical Self-Care

____ Eat regularly (e.g., breakfast, lunch, and dinner)
____ Eat healthily
____ Exercise
____ Get regular medical care for prevention
____ Get medical care when needed
____ Take time off when sick
____ Get massages

____ Dance, swim, walk, run, play sports, sing, or do some other fun physical activity

____ Take time to be sexual—with myself, with a partner

____ Get enough sleep

____ Wear clothes I like

____ Take vacations

____ Other:

Psychological Self-Care

____ Take day trips or mini-vacations

____ Make time away from telephones, email, and the Internet

____ Make time for self-reflection

____ Notice my inner experience—listen to my thoughts, beliefs, attitudes, and feelings

____ Have my own personal psychotherapy

____ Write in a journal

____ Read literature that is unrelated to work

____ Do something at which I am not expert or in charge

____ Attend to minimizing stress in my life

____ Engage my intelligence in a new area, e.g., go to an art show, sports event, and theater

____ Be curious

____ Say no to extra responsibilities sometimes

____ Other:

Emotional Self-Care

____ Spend time with others whose company I enjoy

____ Stay in contact with important people in my life

____ Give myself affirmations, praise myself

____ Love myself

____ Re-read favorite books, re-view favorite movies

_____ Identify comforting activities, objects, people, and
places and seek them out
_____ Allow myself to cry
_____ Find things that make me laugh
_____ Express my outrage in social action, letters, dona-
tions, marches, and protests
_____ Other:

Spiritual Self-Care

_____ Make time for reflection
_____ Spend time in nature
_____ Find a spiritual connection or community
_____ Be open to inspiration
_____ Cherish my optimism and hope
_____ Be aware of non-material aspects of life
_____ Try at times not to be in charge or the expert
_____ Be open to not knowing
_____ Identify what is meaningful to me and notice its
place in my life
_____ Meditate
_____ Pray
_____ Sing
_____ Have experiences of awe
_____ Contribute to causes in which I believe
_____ Read inspirational literature or listen to inspirational
talks, music
_____ Other:

Relationship Self-Care

_____ Schedule regular dates with my partner or spouse
_____ Schedule regular activities with my children
_____ Make time to see friends
_____ Call, check on, or see my relatives

____ Spend time with my companion animals
____ Stay in contact with faraway friends
____ Make time to reply to personal emails and letters; send holiday cards
____ Allow others to do things for me
____ Enlarge my social circle
____ Ask for help when I need it
____ Share a fear, hope, or secret with someone I trust
____ Other:

Workplace or Professional Self-Care

____ Take a break during the workday (e.g., lunch)
____ Take time to chat with co-workers
____ Make quiet time to complete tasks
____ Identify projects or tasks that are exciting and rewarding
____ Set limits with clients and colleagues
____ Balance my caseload so that no one day or part of a day is "too much"
____ Arrange workspace so it is comfortable and comforting
____ Get regular supervision or consultation
____ Negotiate for my needs (benefits, pay raise)
____ Have a peer support group
____ (If relevant) Develop a non-trauma area of professional interest

Overall Balance

____ Strive for balance within my work–life and work day
____ Strive for balance among work, family, relationships, play, and rest

Other Areas of Self-Care That Are Relevant to You

7.3   Burnout

While self-care is important for maintaining well-being, if it does not exist or inadequate, it can lead to a physical and emotional exhaustion known as burnout. According to the World Health Organization, burnout is a syndrome conceptualized as resulting from chronic workplace stress that has not been successfully managed. It is characterized by three dimensions: (1) feelings of energy depletion or exhaustion; (2) increased mental distance from one's job, or feelings of negativism related to one's job; and (3) reduced professional efficacy [4]. Burnout has many variations of definitions, but the similarity of all definitions is that it is developed due to occupational stress. It can occur in any type or level of an occupation or employment. Burnout is a significant issue among healthcare professionals, including NPs.

7.3.1   Burnout in Nurse Practitioners

Burnout among NPs is a growing issue that impacts both individual well-being and patient care. Research by Abraham et al. (2021) found that 25.3% of NPs report burnout, with poor practice environments characterized by high workloads, limited resources, and insufficient administrative support [5]. Conversely, favorable environments with strong NP–physician relations, visibility, autonomy, and support significantly reduce burnout risks by 51–58%.

Similarly, the *2024 Medscape NP Burnout & Depression Report* surveyed 1525 NPs and found that 70% of those NPs experienced burnout or depression, with administrative tasks and poor work–life balance being major factors. Longstanding burnout rates have increased, with 35%

reporting symptoms lasting over two years. One respondent said my "work life balance is nonexistent. I take charting home most nights a week and only have limited time for my interests" [6].

In another study by Kapu et al. (2021), a survey of 1,014 advanced practice registered nurses (APRNs) and physician assistants (PAs), with 94% of respondents being APRNs and 6% PAs, achieving a 43.6% response rate (n = 433), with 76.4% of respondents being NPs [7]. Participants were categorized into groups based on their burnout experiences: currently, previously, or never experienced burnout. Among the 433 respondents, 40.4% (n = 175) reported never experiencing burnout, 33.3% (n = 144) had previously experienced burnout, and 26.3% (n = 114) were currently experiencing burnout. This study highlighted the prevalence of burnout across nurse careers and suggested the need for resilience-building strategies, including self-care and organizational support.

7.3.1.1 Pandemic Effects on Burnout

The coronavirus disease (COVID-19) pandemic drastically heightened burnout among healthcare professionals, particularly those working in frontline and high-stress environments. Both Regestered Nurses (RNs) in hospital settings and NPs in outpatient care have faced unprecedented stressors due to the pandemic. The surge in patient volume, extended working hours, and increased mortality rates during the pandemic placed immense emotional and physical strain on healthcare workers. This surge in demand has led to high levels of burnout, with RNs in particular experiencing significant exhaustion because of frontline roles. A global survey found that 67% of healthcare workers reported burnout during the pandemic, highlighting the intense impact on RNs, who were consistently engaged in crisis management [8].

Beyond the immediate physical and emotional strain, other factors further exacerbated burnout. For example, the constant exposure to critically ill patients, combined with fears of contracting or spreading the virus to family members, significantly increased stress levels. The shortage of personal protective equipment (PPE) during the early stages of the pandemic also contributed to feelings of vulnerability and frustration [8, 9]. These challenges have continued into the post-COVID period, with many healthcare professionals still grappling with the lingering effects of the pandemic. The ongoing pressures facing NPs in outpatient settings, along with the overwhelming demands placed on RNs in hospitals, underscore the need for comprehensive strategies to mitigate burnout and improve the mental and physical well-being of healthcare workers [10, 11].

7.3.1.2   Understanding Burnout Across Healthcare Settings

In addition to the pandemic's impact, burnout in NPs varies across healthcare settings. Primary care, acute care, and rural healthcare each present distinct challenges that contribute to stress and emotional exhaustion. In outpatient primary care, NPs often face high patient loads, administrative responsibilities, and the complexity of managing a wide range of health issues with limited resources, which can lead to feelings of being overwhelmed and emotionally drained [12]. The need to provide continuity of care while juggling clinical duties and administrative tasks intensifies burnout, especially as NPs often lack immediate peer support and may experience professional isolation [13].

In acute care settings, the fast-paced environment, and the high emotional toll of treating critically ill patients further increase stress levels. NPs in these settings frequently encounter burnout due to the intensity of managing severe, life-threatening cases, which adds to the emotional burden [14, 15]. Meanwhile, NPs working in rural healthcare face unique challenges, such as professional isolation, resource scarcity, and the need to address diverse medical issues with limited support, all of which contribute to heightened burnout [16, 17]. These varied settings underscore the importance of addressing burnout in ways that are tailored to the specific pressures NPs face in their respective environments.

7.4   Compassion Fatigue

Burnout can affect professionals across many fields, but compassion fatigue is specific to healthcare and human services. Compassion fatigue is commonly defined as "the convergence of secondary traumatic stress and cumulative burnout, a state of physical and mental exhaustion caused by a depleted ability to cope with one's everyday environment" [18]. Another broader definition describes it as "a state of exhaustion and dysfunction biologically, psychotically, and socially, as a result of prolonged exposure to compassion stress and all it invokes" [19]. These definitions highlight the complex, multifaceted nature of compassion fatigue and its impact on healthcare providers. Although not included in the DSM-5, compassion fatigue shares similarities with post-traumatic stress disorder and secondary traumatic stress. It occurs when healthcare providers are repeatedly exposed to the trauma and suffering of others. Like burnout, symptoms may include fatigue, helplessness, emotional numbness, or being preoccupied with others' trauma.

7.4.1　The Impact on Nurse Practitioners

Compassion fatigue can occur with the continuous act of caring for others, especially in high-stress settings. This can drain NPs both emotionally and mentally. Over time, this emotional depletion can manifest as physical and psychological exhaustion, reduced empathy, and a decreased ability to provide quality care. Studies have shown that prolonged exposure to compassion stress can lead to cognitive impairments, emotional numbness, and difficulty connecting with patients on a personal level [18]. As a result, NPs may experience a diminished capacity to perform their jobs effectively, which not only impacts patient care but also leads to dissatisfaction with their professional roles.

Furthermore, compassion fatigue can exacerbate feelings of professional isolation, especially in fields where peer support is limited. NPs in rural settings, for example, may face the additional challenge of working without immediate access to colleagues who can provide emotional or professional support. Without adequate coping mechanisms and support systems, compassion fatigue can contribute to burnout, which has a direct negative impact on job retention and patient outcomes.

7.5　Strength in the Storm: A Personal NP Story

By Alyssa Sonneborn FNP-BC

As healthcare providers, we aim to care for and treat our patients, hoping to see their well-being improve. Yet, during the COVID pandemic, no matter our efforts, no matter how hard we worked, or how far we went, it was not enough. As a nurse, much of my job satisfaction came from seeing patients improve, so when, despite our dedication, patients continued to suffer, it created a defeating cycle. In the Intensive Care Unit (ICU), I found myself in an endless routine, where nearly every patient who arrived would likely not leave, and we became like a well-oiled machine, anticipating the rapid decline that became an expectation. Each shift brought exponential challenges, as I knew the patients I cared for and spoke with would likely face intubation and may never come off life support.

The height of the pandemic was even more isolating for patients, as visitor restrictions meant that families could not be present—particularly in the ICU, where aerosolization risks were highest. Nurses became the strength, love, and support those patients needed. We face Timed families at the end of life, and I often cried with them, sitting beside their loved ones as they succumbed to one of the most frustrating viruses I have ever encountered.

During this intense time, I was also in graduate school to become an NP, which added another layer of stress. I was also navigating a personal separation and adjusting to being a single mom. Every day, I am thankful for the support of my colleagues, classmates, and family during that time. They gave me the strength to push forward with the positive energy my patients so desperately needed. Yet, the lack of positive outcomes and patients' struggles weighed heavily on me, leading to burnout that has progressed over the years. I am still grappling with this. I eventually left the hospital setting, hoping to rediscover my passion for healthcare.

The pandemic will never be forgotten. Specific patients and families are etched in my memory forever. I wouldn't be where I am today without the unwavering support from those around me.

7.5.1   Assessing and Addressing Compassion Fatigue

Compassion fatigue is a significant and growing concern for healthcare professionals, particularly NPs. It manifests as emotional and physical exhaustion, often resulting from the high demands of caring for patients in distress. Addressing compassion fatigue requires a multifaceted approach, with assessments serving as a critical first step. One of the most used tools is the Professional Quality of Life (ProQOL) survey, which distinguishes between compassion fatigue, burnout, and secondary traumatic stress. This free resource identifies compassion fatigue and helps develop effective coping strategies [18].

The ProQOL survey includes questions designed to assess the emotional experiences of healthcare professionals. It focuses on three key areas: compassion satisfaction, burnout, and secondary traumatic stress. Respondents answer questions about their levels of satisfaction from helping others, feelings of exhaustion, and stress, with responses rated on a scale from 1 to 5. The results offer insights into the levels of compassion satisfaction, burnout, and secondary trauma, providing healthcare workers with a better understanding of their emotional well-being. A study by Glover-Stief, Jannen, and Cohn (2021) involving 208 NPs revealed that mindfulness practices were associated with reduced burnout and compassion fatigue. Additionally, the study found that strong support from co-workers and family members significantly mitigated the effects of these challenges. These findings highlight the importance of both internal coping strategies, such as mindfulness, and external support systems in managing compassion fatigue [20]. Although the NP may know these strategies, their organization must value and support addressing this issue.

7.5.1.1 Workplace Support

The research underscores the critical need for robust support systems within the workplace to help NPs manage compassion fatigue effectively. Education provided by administrators regarding the symptoms and effects of compassion fatigue can empower healthcare professionals to recognize and address this condition in themselves and their colleagues. Equally vital is fostering a supportive community among co-workers, which can ease the emotional burden and reduce the impact of compassion fatigue on patient care.

The workplace can also offer interventional programs such as mindfulness, yoga, and meditation. These have been shown to alleviate symptoms of burnout. In emotionally demanding specialties such as palliative care or hospice, offering specialized training, self-care resources, and bereavement programs can reduce stress and promote well-being [21]. Without these essential supports, compassion fatigue will continue to hinder healthcare professionals' ability to provide high-quality care, ultimately affecting patient outcomes.

7.6   Resilience

While addressing compassion fatigue is critical, developing resilience offers a more proactive and sustainable approach to managing the stress and emotional demands of healthcare. Resilience is a broad concept that encompasses many aspects of life, including personal, social, and occupational dimensions. For nurses, however, resilience plays a particularly vital role in sustaining their careers. According to Cooper et al. (2021), "Resiliency is a complex and dynamic process that, when present and sustained, enables nurses to positively adapt to workplace stressors, avoid psychological harm, and continue to provide safe, high-quality patient care" [22]. NPs must develop the capacity to cope with and thrive in stressful environments. Understanding resilience is crucial not only for NPs but also for their managers, as it directly supports their ability to manage stressors and provide quality care.

Research has consistently shown that resilience is a key factor in NPs' effectiveness as healthcare providers. Studies indicate that those with higher levels of resilience report lower burnout rates and greater job satisfaction [20].

Several strategies offer a structured and mindful approach to building resilience [23]. Goal setting is important for maintaining focus and momentum, especially during challenging times. For example, simplifying tasks and aiming to accomplish "one task a day" helps prevent feelings of overwhelm. Cognitive-behavioral strategies are also essential, focusing on managing thinking traps, boosting self-efficacy, and employing goal-directed thinking to tackle adversity. Additionally, emotional support plays a foundational role; seeking help and cultivating supportive relationships are crucial for sustaining resilience. Finally, developing self-efficacy and applying hope theory—building confidence in one's ability to overcome challenges while maintaining hope—are essential for perseverance and long-term resilience.

7.6.1   Case Study for Application

Omar, a Family Nurse Practitioner (FNP) in a busy primary care clinic, has been practicing for five years. He began his career with enthusiasm, eager to make a difference in his patients' lives. However, over time, he began to feel overwhelmed by the increasing workload, long hours, and the emotional demands of caring for chronically ill patients. The clinic also faced staff shortages, which meant Omar had to take on more patients than usual, often seeing over 25 patients a day.

Omar started to experience physical symptoms like headaches and fatigue. Emotionally, he felt detached from his work, struggling to find the compassion he once had for the patients. These feelings culminated in burnout, making him question whether he could continue in the profession.

Despite these challenges, Omar recognized the need to make a change before her burnout worsened. He began to explore resilience strategies, seeking out mentorship, prioritizing self-care, and setting boundaries at work.

Identification of Resilience Strategies (For Discussion):

1. **Mentorship and support:** Omar reached out to a senior NP who had gone through a similar experience and received guidance on navigating burnout. This type of mentorship helped him feel less isolated and provided him with practical advice.
2. **Setting boundaries:** Omar started to set clearer boundaries at work, learning to say no to excessive overtime and taking time off when needed. He also worked with the clinic manager to create a more manageable schedule, reducing the number of patients he saw each day.
3. **Mindfulness and self-care:** To address the physical symptoms, Omar began practicing mindfulness meditation off a phone application and made time for physical activity, which helped manage stress. He also prioritized regular sleep and took time to disconnect from work during weekends.

4. **Seeking professional help:** Recognizing that his emotional health was at stake, Omar sought counseling, which provided him with tools to manage the emotional exhaustion.

Reflection Questions:

1. How would you address the physical symptoms Omar experienced?
2. What resilience strategies would you prioritize if you were in Omar's situation?

7.6.2 Strategies to Combat Burnout and Enhance Resilience

Resilience plays an important role in preventing burnout and promoting long-term well-being. Exploring strategies that healthcare professionals can implement to strengthen their resilience would be helpful. This will help maintain the ability to provide high-quality care in the face of adversity. Addressing burnout requires understanding its multifaceted nature and implementing tailored strategies to support the NPs in different settings.

Effective approaches to combat burnout and enhance resilience include promoting self-care practices, fostering supportive organizational cultures, and providing opportunities for professional development and leadership [11]. These measures can enhance resilience, job satisfaction, and overall well-being among NPs. This ultimately can lead to improved patient outcomes. For example, encouraging self-care and work–life balance helps manage stress, while supportive workplace environments and peer support can mitigate feelings of professional isolation. Additionally, continuous professional development and leadership opportunities can empower NPs, reducing burnout and improving job satisfaction [7, 24].

Harwood, Crandall, and LeFuentes (2024) found in their quantitative cross-sectional study of NPs, 80.9% had moderate to high levels of burnout and minimal job satisfaction [25]. To address the alarming levels of burnout, it was recommended implementing structured interventions focused on resilience-building strategies and stress management programs. They suggested that hospital leadership could enhance support by offering regular workshops on mindfulness, coping mechanisms, and time management tailored specifically for NPs. Additionally, they advocated for the development of peer support networks and mentorship programs. Overall, hospital leaders needed to take a more proactive role in promoting education in self-care and resiliency, which could contribute to greater job satisfaction and reduce turnover.

Shanafelt and Noseworthy (2017) outlined nine organizational strategies to promote engagement and reduce burnout, emphasizing the importance of executive leadership in fostering a supportive work environment [11]. The first step is acknowledging the problem by openly recognizing the presence of burnout within the organization. Transparency fosters an environment where employees feel comfortable discussing their challenges and paves the way for meaningful interventions. Alongside this, recognizing leadership behaviors that promote respect and support is crucial, as leaders significantly influence the workplace atmosphere. By cultivating leadership styles that encourage empathy and engagement, organizations can directly reduce burnout rates.

Additionally, developing targeted interventions tailored to the specific needs of staff can provide practical support. This may include stress-reduction workshops, mentoring programs, or wellness initiatives. Building a strong sense of community is also vital; cultivating collaboration and social support through team-building activities can alleviate feel-ings of isolation and improve morale. Strategic recognition, such as using rewards, can further enhance job satisfaction by acknowledging employees' hard work with initiatives like employee-of-the-month programs or bonuses.

Furthermore, ensuring that the organization's actions are aligned with its core values can foster a sense of purpose among employees, helping them reconnect with their roles. Promoting work–life balance through flexible scheduling and manageable workloads is essential to prevent burnout. Providing self-care resources, such as mindfulness pro-grams and counseling services, equips employees with tools to manage stress and improve well-being. Finally, support-ing organizational science by utilizing evidence-based prac-tices and regularly surveying employee well-being allows organizations to stay proactive in preventing burnout and fostering employee engagement. Through these strategies, leaders can create a healthier, more resilient workforce.

7.7   Emotional Intelligence

Another skill that is essential for healthcare providers to have is emotional intelligence (EI). However, EI is the ability to recognize, understand, manage, and influence one's own emotions [26]. EI helps manage personal stress and avoid burnout. The main components of EI are self-awareness, self-regulation, motivation, empathy, and social skills. EI equips healthcare providers with the tools to han-dle demanding situations effectively, contributing to a more supportive and patient-centered care environment.

Othman et al. (2024) explored the relationship between EI, job satisfaction, and organizational commitment among nurse managers [27]. The findings reveal that EI positively influences both job satisfaction and organizational commitment, with nurse managers exhibiting moderate to high levels of commitment and job satisfaction. These managers reported more control over emotions and balanced response to challenges in the workplace. The results suggest that training in EI can be a strategic approach to improve healthcare outcomes by enhancing job satisfaction and commitment to an organization (Othman et al., 2024).

7.7.1 Components of Emotional Intelligence

The core components of EI are self-awareness, self-regulation, motivation, empathy, and social skills. These components play a vital role in fostering resilience and enhancing patient interactions. Self-awareness is the ability to recognize and understand your emotions, thoughts, and behaviors, and how they affect both yourself and others, enabling you to reflect on and manage your responses [26]. Self-regulation refers to the ability to control or redirect disruptive emotions and impulses, maintaining composure and adapting to changing circumstances. Motivation entails a strong drive to achieve goals, commitment to patient care, and a passion for the profession, leading to increased resilience and perseverance. Empathy allows healthcare providers to connect with patients, build trust, and provide compassionate care. Social skills enable effective communication, conflict resolution, and teamwork.

7.7.2 Impact of Emotional Intelligence

Emotional intelligence is suggested to have a significant impact on healthcare outcomes, particularly in enhancing patient-centered care and job satisfaction [28]. EI may improve communication, help professionals better understand patient emotions, and foster more compassionate care, potentially improving the patient experience. EI is essential for healthcare providers as it significantly impacts their effectiveness and patient care quality [26]. There is a relationship between EI and various factors such as stress, coping strategies, well-being, and academic performance [29]. Conducted with 130 students in the UK, the study found that higher EI was positively related to well-being, problem-focused coping, and perceived nursing competency, while it was negatively related to perceived stress. When EI is higher, one is better equipped to handle stress though coping strategies. This improves the overall well-being. Enhancing EI in nursing schools and other academic settings can benefit the healthcare providers mental health and overall performance.

7.7.3   Improving Emotional Intelligence

Improving EI is a valuable approach for enhancing personal and professional effectiveness. By developing a deeper understanding of one's emotions and strengthening interpersonal skills, individuals can better manage stress, build resilient relationships, and improve communication [30]. Focusing on core EI components, such as self-awareness, self-regulation, empathy, motivation, and social skills, offers a pathway to greater well-being and success in various environments, especially in healthcare.

7.7.3.1   Self-Awareness

Self-awareness can be enhanced by journaling, reflecting on daily experiences and emotions [29]. Writing down moments where there were strong emotions and analyzing what triggered those feelings can help identify patterns and triggers. In addition to journaling, meditation practice can help one be more in tune with emotions. Observing thoughts and emotions can identify how emotions can influence behavior. Another way to be more aware is gathering feedback from peers and friends to help uncover any behavior blind spots and make way for improvement.

7.7.3.2   Self-Regulation

Some effective self-regulation techniques include pausing before reacting, identifying emotional triggers, and developing personalized coping strategies [30]. In emotionally charged situations, practicing a brief pause, and taking a few deep breaths can help manage impulsive reactions, allowing individuals to respond in a calm and composed manner. When feelings of overwhelm arise, it is important to recognize and document the emotional triggers involved, which can help in preparing for similar situations in the future. Coping strategies vary from person to person, so it is essential to identify stress management techniques that work best for the individual. These may include activities like walking, deep breathing, knitting, or talking to a trusted friend. By employing these techniques, individuals can better manage their emotional responses and improve overall well-being.

7.7.3.3   Empathy

Building empathy supports EI by enhancing one's ability to understand and connect with others on an emotional level. Empathy can be developed through active listening, asking open-ended questions, and perspective-taking. Practicing active listening involves fully focusing on the speaker during conversations by maintaining eye contact, nodding, and paraphrasing what the other person says. This shows that you value their perspective and emotions. Asking open-ended questions, such as "How do you feel about this situation?" or "What can I do to support you?" encourages others to share their thoughts and feelings, allowing you to gain a deeper understanding of their emotions. Additionally, perspective-taking, or putting yourself in someone else's shoes, helps build empathy by considering their experiences and responding with compassion.

7.7.3.4   Motivation

To build motivation, it is important to set both personal and professional goals that are clear, achievable, and inspiring. By keeping track of your progress and celebrating small wins along the way, you can maintain a sense of accomplishment and stay driven. When faced with challenges, maintaining a positive outlook is key; focus on solutions rather than problems by reframing negative thoughts into more constructive ones. As a leader, you can also motivate others by leading through example. Demonstrating enthusiasm and a strong work ethic shows your team that you are committed to achieving organizational goals, which can inspire them to follow your lead and stay motivated as well.

7.7.3.5   Social Skills

Developing strong social skills is essential for building effective relationships and enhancing EI among healthcare providers. Improving communication involves expressing thoughts clearly and concisely, both in writing and verbally, while remaining receptive to feedback and input from others. In conflict situations, constructive approaches— such as addressing issues directly and calmly, finding common ground, and collaborating on mutually beneficial solutions—can be effective. Additionally, investing time in building relationships with colleagues through personal connections, participation in social events, sharing ideas, and collaborating on projects fosters a more cohesive and collaborative work environment.

Combating burnout and enhancing resilience in healthcare professionals, particularly NPs, requires a multifaceted approach that integrates both individual and organizational strategies. Research emphasizes that promoting self-care practices, fostering supportive workplace environments, and providing opportunities for professional development are some strategies to address burnout and improve resilience [11, 25]. Moreover, the role of EI is also highlighted as a significant factor in reducing stress and improving job satisfaction and patient care outcomes [26, 28]. By focusing on both internal skills such as self-regulation and empathy, and external supports, NPs can develop a robust toolkit for managing stress and avoiding burnout. Work initiatives such as mindfulness programs, work–life balance policies, and leadership training can empower NPs to remain engaged and effective in their roles. Building resilience and combating burnout require a comprehensive approach that incorporates both personal development and organizational responsibility. By adopting these strategies, healthcare systems can better support NPs in maintaining their mental health, job satisfaction, and ability to provide high-quality patient care, even in the most demanding environments.

Assignment #1: Reflective Journal on Burnout Experiences

Goal: To enhance self-awareness and understanding of burnout through personal reflection and analysis.

Objectives:

1. Identify personal experiences and signs of burnout.
2. Analyze the factors contributing to burnout in healthcare settings.
3. Evaluate coping strategies and their effectiveness in managing burnout.
4. Create a personal action plan to mitigate burnout and promote resilience.

Instructions:

1. Write a weekly reflective journal entry for one to two weeks.
2. In each entry, describe a situation where you felt stressed, overwhelmed, or burned out.
3. Reflect on the contributing factors to your feelings of burnout.
4. Discuss the strategies you used to cope with these feelings.
5. Evaluate the effectiveness of these strategies.
6. Develop a personal action plan to prevent and manage burnout, incorporating lessons learned from your reflections.

Rubric

Criteria	Exemplary (10 points)	Proficient (8 points)	Adequate (6 points)	Needs Improvement (4 points)	Unsatisfactory (2 points)
Identification of burnout experiences	Thorough identification of burnout experiences	Clear identification of burnout experiences	General identification of burnout experiences	Unclear identification of burnout experiences	Minimal or no identification of burnout experiences
Analysis of contributing factors	In-depth analysis of contributing factors/connections to burnout	Good analysis of contributing factors with connections to burnout	Basic analysis of contributing factors with limited to none connections to burnout	Limited analysis of contributing factors with no connections to burnout	Minimal or no analysis of contributing factors
Evaluation of coping strategies	Comprehensive evaluation of coping strategies with examples	Good evaluation of coping strategies with examples	Basic evaluation of coping strategies with examples	Limited evaluation of coping strategies with little or no examples	Minimal or no evaluation of coping strategies
Development of a personal action plan	Well-developed, actionable, and realistic personal action plan	Actionable and realistic personal action plan	Basic personal action plan with some actionable steps	Limited personal action plan with few actionable steps	Minimal or no personal action plan
Clarity and depth of reflection	Exceptionally clear and deep reflection	Clear and thoughtful reflection	General and adequate reflection	Unclear or superficial reflection	Minimal or no reflection

Total: 50 points

Assignment #2:   Case Study Analysis on Resilience and Burnout

Goal: To apply theoretical knowledge of resilience to a real-world scenario in healthcare.

Objectives:

1. Analyze a case study to identify resilience strategies.
2. Apply resilience-building techniques to hypothetical scenarios.
3. Synthesize insights to improve personal and professional resilience.

Instructions:

Read the case study and identify some resilience strategies employed by the individual to cope with burnout. Be specific. Discuss how these resilience strategies can be applied to your own practice as an NP, highlighting any insights gained from the case studies.

Scenario:

A new NP, Genevieve, just started working in a rural healthcare setting. Genevieve is passionate about helping underserved populations but quickly becomes overwhelmed by the demands of rural practice. The clinic is understaffed, and Genevieve is expected to handle both acute and chronic care for a diverse patient population. With limited resources, Genevieve starts working long hours and takes work home, causing a strain on personal relationships and leaving little time for self-care.

Within a few months, Genevieve begins to experience burnout symptoms, including fatigue, irritability, and emotional exhaustion. Recognizing these signs early, she decides to take proactive steps to build resilience.

Resilience Strategies for Genevieve: Give Examples of Each Item Below and Be Specific

1. **Peer support group**
2. **Time management and delegation**
3. **Developing a wellness routine**
4. **Boundary setting**.

Application of Resilience Strategies to Personal Practice:

As an NP, these resilience strategies can be directly applied to practice.

Write three to four paragraphs on how these strategies can be applied to practice. Give specific actionable insights to apply.

(continued)

Rubric

Criteria	Exemplary (9–10 points)	Proficient (7–8 points)	Satisfactory (5–6 points)	Needs Improvement (0–4 points)	Points
Identification of Resilience Strategies	Clearly identifies all key resilience strategies used by Omar and Genevieve, providing detailed and specific examples	Identifies most resilience strategies with some relevant examples, but lacks depth in a few areas	Identifies some resilience strategies, but examples are vague or incomplete	Fails to identify key resilience strategies or examples are inaccurate or missing	/10
Application of Resilience Strategies to Practice	Provides a thoughtful and detailed discussion on how resilience strategies can be applied to personal practice, with specific, actionable insights	Discusses application to practice with mostly specific insights, though some areas could use more depth	Offers some application of resilience strategies to practice, but insights are general or lack detail	Fails to adequately apply resilience strategies to practice, or the discussion is unclear or incomplete	/10

Total Points: 20

Assignment #3: Emotional Intelligence Workshop Development

Goal: To design and implement a workshop aimed at enhancing EI among NPs.

Objectives:

1. Define EI and its importance in healthcare.
2. Design activities and exercises to develop EI skills.
3. Implement the workshop with a peer group.
4. Evaluate the effectiveness of the workshop and suggest improvements.

Instructions:

1. Research and define the concept of EI in healthcare.
2. Design a 2–4-hour workshop that includes activities and exercises to develop EI skills.
3. Implement the workshop with a group of peers.
4. Collect feedback from participants on the effectiveness of the workshop.
5. Write a report summarizing the workshop design, implementation, participant feedback, and suggestions for improvement.

Rubric

Definition and importance of EI (5 points)
Design of workshop activities and exercises (5 points)
Implementation of the workshop (5 points)
Collection and analysis of participant feedback (5 points)
Report summary and suggestions for improvement (5 points)

Total: 25 points

7.8 Conclusion

Self-care is no longer an add-on or a luxury activity for the healthcare profession. Healthcare is in a crisis with fewer healthcare providers, the need for more rural care and specialized care, a decrease the number of nurses and support staff. To support healthcare workers to remain professionally healthy and to avoid burnout and compassion fatigue, leaders in healthcare need to focus on self-care and implement programs to promote. Individuals in healthcare also need to take responsibility for themselves and design a self-care plan and provide themselves the opportunity to enhance their resilience and reduce their stressors.

> **"You can't pour from an empty cup. Take care of yourself first."—Unknown**

Other Self-Care Resources
Self-Care Tool Website
In order to understand self-care and to learn more information about how to implement activities such as breathing, sleep routines, grounding, physical activity, journaling, and more, go to this website: https://proqol.org/self-care-tools-1

Applications for Self-Care
Apps are a way to have easy access to tools for self-care and to have a way to keep a record of what you are doing daily for yourself.

1. **Insight Timer**
   Features: Thousands of free guided meditations, including guided imagery exercises, sleep aids, and mindfulness practices. It also has a community feature for support.

Cost: Free with optional in-app purchases and a premium membership for additional features.

Website: https://insighttimer.com/

2. **Smiling Mind**

Features: Mindfulness and meditation programs designed by psychologists and educators, tailored for different age groups and needs.

Cost: Free.

Website: https://www.smilingmind.com.au/

3. **Calm**

Features: Guided meditations, sleep stories, breathing exercises, and relaxation music. Calm offers specific programs for stress reduction and relaxation.

Cost: Free basic version with a limited selection of content; premium subscription for full access.

Website: https://www.calm.com/

4. **Headspace**

Features: Guided meditations, mindfulness exercises, sleep aids, and programs focused on stress, anxiety, and sleep.

Cost: Free basic version with a limited selection of content; premium subscription for full access. Often offers discounted rates for students and healthcare professionals.

Website: https://www.headspace.com/

5. **University of California, Los Angeles (UCLA) Mindful**

Features: Guided meditations and mindfulness exercises developed by the UCLA Mindful Awareness Research Center.

Cost: Free.

Website: https://www.uclahealth.org/uclamindful

How to Create a Self-Care Plan for Nurses

Take the following steps to develop a plan for self-care:

Step 1

The first step to crafting a reasonable self-care plan is self-reflection and self-assessment. Where are you currently with self-care? You may wish to assess the following areas of your life:

- Physical
- Mental
- Spiritual
- Personal
- Economic
- Psychological

Step 2

Identify opportunities for growth. What areas do you see deficits? Are you not paying attention to your spiritual side?

Step 3

Decide which interventions you need to implement. Examples include:

- **Physical**: Get regular health screenings, eat clean and nutritious meals, maintain a healthy weight, and exercise.
- **Mental**: Use relaxation and imagery techniques. Focus attention away from fear-based, negative thought patterns and become more open to life-affirming information and patterns of thought. Seek books and groups that promote joy, and pursue counseling if necessary.
- **Spiritual**: Engage in activities that develop your higher self. This could be accomplished via a religious

affiliation, but it does not have to be. Practice meditation or yoga and say positive affirmations.

- **Personal**: Engage in truthful and caring self-reflection regarding your communication with others. Identify both the cohesiveness and the disharmony in your relationships. Strive to be aware of the effect both have on family and friends. Nurture important relationships.
- **Economic**: Live within your means. Take the steps necessary to balance your economic health. Sometimes, less is more.
- **Psychological**: Embrace your creativity and play. Identify what stimulates your mind and invest time into these activities.

(Purdue Global, 2019)

Daily Affirmations

Daily validation and affirming can help change the way we think and respond to situations. It can generally make us feel more positive about ourselves and our world.

1. I am ready.
2. My efforts help me succeed.
3. I can make a real difference.
4. My hard work will pay off.
5. I am strong.
6. I have the power to make the right choices for me.
7. I have faith in my abilities.
8. I got this.
9. I am grateful for what I can do.
10. I am happy to be me.
11. My goals are achievable.
12. I am confident.

13. I will be kind to myself today.
14. I am on the right path for me.
15. I deserve love in my life.
16. I will take action to accomplish my goals.
17. I will celebrate the progress I'm making to reach my goals.
18. I will look for the good in things.
19. I am always learning.
20. I trust myself.
21. I will try new things.
22. I will turn negative thoughts into positive ones.
23. I will accept myself as I am.
24. I love myself.
25. I will make time for what brings me joy.
26. I am powerful.
27. I believe in myself.
28. It's OK for me to have fun.
29. My possibilities are endless.
30. I am well-rested and full of energy.
31. I am relaxed and at peace.
32. I am strong in mind, body, and spirit.
33. My life is a gift.
34. I deserve love and happiness.
35. I care for myself.
36. Healthy food fuels my body.
37. Today, I will take steps to reach my goals.
38. I give myself room to make mistakes and grow.
39. I will find moments of joy today.
40. I embrace my power.

Kaiser Permanente. (2023). Forty positive affirmations for better self-care. https://healthy.kaiserpermanente. org/health-wellness/healtharticle.40-positive-affirmations

References

1. Halm, M. (2017). The role of mindfulness in enhancing self-care for nurses. *Am. J. Crit. Care* 26 (4): 344–348. https://doi.org/10.4037/ajcc2017589.
2. Mason, W. (2019). The Importance of Self-Care for Nurses and How to Put a Plan in Place | Purdue Global | (accessed 27 April 2023).
3. Butler, L. D. (2010). Self-care assessment. http://www.ballarat.edu.au/aasp/student/sds/self_care_assess.shtml (Original work adapted from Saakvitne, K. W., Pearlman, L. A., & Staff of TSI/CAAP. (1996). Transforming the pain: A workbook on vicarious traumatization. Norton).
4. World Health Organization (2019). Burn-out: an occupations phenomenon. https://www.who.int/news/item/28-05-2019-burn-out-an-occupational-phenomenon-international-classification-of-diseases (accessed 28 May 2019).
5. Abraham, C.M., Zheng, K., Norful, A.A. et al. (2021). Primary care practice environment and burnout among nurse practitioners. *J. Nurse Pract.* 17 (2): 157–162. https://doi.org/10.1016/j.nurpra.2020.11.009.
6. Medscape (2024). A Silent Struggle: Nurse Practitioner Burnout & Depression Report.
7. Kapu, A.N., Borg Card, E., Jackson, H. et al. (2021). Assessing and addressing practitioner burnout: results from an advanced practice registered nurse health and well-being study. *J. Am. Assoc. Nurse Pract.* 33 (1): 38–48. https://doi.org/10.1097/JXX.0000000000000324.
8. Morgantini, L.A., Naha, U., Wang, H. et al. (2020). Factors contributing to healthcare professional burnout during the COVID-19 pandemic: a rapid turnaround global survey. *PLoS One* 15 (9): e0238217.
9. Kisely, S., Warren, N., McMahon, L. et al. (2020). Occurrence, prevention, and management of the psychological effects of emerging virus outbreaks on healthcare workers: rapid review and meta-analysis. *BMJ* 369: m1642.
10. Maslach, C. and Leiter, M.P. (2016). Understanding the burnout experience: recent research and its implications for psychiatry. *World Psychiatry* 15 (2): 103–111.

11. Shanafelt, T.D. and Noseworthy, J.H. (2017). Executive leadership and physician well-being: nine organizational strategies to promote engagement and reduce burnout. *Mayo. Clin. Proc.* 92 (1): 129–146.

12. Bodenheimer, T. and Sinsky, C. (2014). From triple to quadruple aim: care of the patient requires care of the provider. *Ann. Fam. Med.* 12 (6): 573–576.

13. Spinelli, W.M., Fernstrom, K.M., Galentino, R., and Bohman, B. (2016). Factors associated with burnout during residency training: a systematic review. *J. Grad. Med. Educ.* 8 (4): 516–527.

14. Embriaco, N., Papazian, L., Kentish-Barnes, N. et al. (2007). Burnout syndrome among critical care healthcare workers. *Curr. Opin. Crit. Care* 13 (5): 482–488.

15. Moss, M., Good, V.S., Gozal, D. et al. (2016). An official critical care societies collaborative statement: burnout syndrome in critical care health-care professionals: a call for action. *Am. J. Respir. Crit. Care Med.* 194 (1): 106–113.

16. Andrews, D.R. and Wan, T.T.H. (2009). The importance of mental health to the experience of job strain: an evidence-guided approach to improve retention. *J. Nurs. Manag.* 17 (3): 340–351.

17. Kulig, J.C., Kilpatrick, K., Moffitt, P., and Zimmer, L. (2012). Rural and remote nursing practice: an analysis of policy documents. *Aust. J. Rural HealthAustralian Journal of Rural Health* 20 (5): 235–239.

18. Cocker, F. and Joss, N. (2016). Compassion fatigue among healthcare, emergency and community service workers: a systematic review. *Int. J. Environ. Res. Public Health* 13 (6): 618.

19. Figley, C. (1995). Compassion fatigue as secondary traumatic stress disorder: an overview. In: *Compassion Fatigue: Coping with Secondary Stress Disorder in Those Who Treat the Traumatised* (ed. C.R. Figley). Bristol, UK: Brunner/Mazel.

20. Glover-Stief, M., Jannen, S., and Cohn, T. (2021). An exploratory descriptive study of compassion fatigue and compassion satisfaction: examining potential risk and protective factors in advanced nurse practitioners. *J. Am. Assoc. Nurse Pract.* 33 (2): 143–149. 10.1097/JXX.0000000000000357.

21. Cross, L.A. (2019). Compassion fatigue in palliative care nursing: a conceptanalysis.*J.Hosp.Palliat.Nurs.*21(1):21–28.https://doi.

org/10.1097/NJH.0000000000000477. PMID: 30608916; PMCID: PMC6343956.

22. Cooper, A.L., Brown, J.A., and Leslie, G.D. (2021). Nurse resilience for clinical practice: an integrative review. *J. Adv. Nurs.* 77 (6): 2623–2640.

23. Hone, L. C. (2016). Understanding and measuring wellbeing. Doctoral thesis. Auckland University of Technology. AUT Research Repository.

24. Maslach, C. and Jackson, S.E. (1981). The measurement of experienced burnout. *J. Occup. Behav.* 2 (2): 99–113.

25. Harwood, L., Crandall, J., and LeFuentes, A. (2024). Burnout, resilience and job satisfaction in acute care nurse practitioners. *Nurs. Leadersh. (Tor Ont).* 37 (1): 29–51. https://doi.org/10.12927/cjnl.2024.27357. PMID: 39087272.

26. Cherry, M.G., Fletcher, I., O'Sullivan, H., and Dornan, T. (2019). Emotional intelligence in medical education: a critical review. *Med. Educ.* 48 (5): 468–478. https://doi.org/10.1111/medu.12324.

27. Othman, M.I., Khalifeh, A., Oweidat, I., and Nashwan, A.J. (2024). The relationship between emotional intelligence, job satisfaction, and organizational commitment among first-line nurse managers in Qatar. *J. Nurs. Manag.* 2024: 5114659.

28. Birks, Y.F. and Watt, I.S. (2007). Emotional intelligence and patient-centered care. *J. R. Soc. Med.* 100 (8): 368–374. https://doi.org/10.1258/jrsm.100.8.368.

29. Por, J., Barriball, L., Fitzpatrick, J., and Roberts, J. (2011). Emotional intelligence: its relationship to stress, coping, well-being and professional performance in nursing students. *Nurse. Educ. Today* 31 (8): 855–860. https://doi.org/10.1016/j.nedt.2010.12.023.Epub. PMID: 21292360.

30. Landry, L. (2021). *Emotional Intelligence Skills: What They Are & How to Develop Them.* Harvard Business School Online https://online.hbs.edu/blog/post/emotional-intelligence-skills.

Chapter 8

Identifying Opportunities for Advancement

Sara L. Gleasman-DeSimone, PhD, ANP-C

Le Moyne College, Graduate Nursing Department, Syracuse, NY, USA

The Leap of Faith
Colleen Zogby, FNP-C, PhD Candidate
Le Moyne College, Syracuse, NY, USA

Entrepreneurship in Nursing
Theresa Setter, APRN-BC, DCNP
Revitalize Dermatology & Aesthetics, Fayetteville, NY, USA

Nurse Practitioner: Transition Guide, First Edition. Sara L. Gleasman-DeSimone.
© 2025 John Wiley & Sons, Inc. Published 2025 by John Wiley & Sons, Inc.

Snapshot of AI in Healthcare
Charles P. DeSimone, PhD
Upstate Medical University, Syracuse, NY, USA

Fostering the Future
Deborah Clarey, FNP-C, RFNA
Mohawk Valley Health System, Oneida, NY, USA

Chapter Highlights

Continuing Education
Recertification
Doctor of Nursing Practice
Entrepreneurship
Outcome Measures
Interprofessional Education
Artificial Intelligence

8.1   Introduction

Nurse practitioners (NPs) are at the forefront of delivering high-quality, patient-centered care in today's rapidly evolving healthcare environment. As the demands on healthcare systems become more complex, NPs must extend their clinical expertise and develop a broad range of skills to tackle emerging challenges. This chapter explores foundational topics such as continuing education (CE) and recertification, as well as advanced innovations like integrating artificial intelligence (AI) into practice. It also highlights the growing importance of entrepreneurial thinking and the global expansion of NP roles.

"Every moment is a fresh beginning."—T. S. Eliot

> # Objectives with Mapping to 2021 AACN Masters Essentials
>
> Identify continuing education and certification opportunities. Domain 10: Personal, Professional, and Leadership Development
>
> Analyze the role of the Doctor of Nursing Practice (DNP) degree in preparing NPs for leadership and evidence-based care implementation. Domain 8: Clinical Judgment and Evidence-Based Practice
>
> Understand entrepreneurial skills to design innovative healthcare solutions. Domain 6: Interprofessional Partnerships
>
> Use HEDIS performance measures to implement quality improvement initiatives. Domain 3: Population Health; Domain 7: Quality and Safety
>
> Design strategies to integrate Interprofessional Education (IPE) into clinical practice. Domain 6: Interprofessional Partnerships
>
> Examine the applications and limitations of AI technologies. Domain 2: Informatics and Healthcare Technologies

8.2   Elevating Practice

8.2.1   Continuing Education

In the evolving field of healthcare, staying up to date is important for delivering the best possible patient care. NPs must embrace lifelong learning as they move through their professional journey. The first year of practice is a valuable time for NPs to explore CE opportunities such as workshops, conferences, online courses, and specialty certifications. While CE focuses on expanding knowledge and refining skills, recertification serves as a formal mechanism to ensure NPs maintain their competencies.

8.2.1.1 Recertification

Recertification ensures that NPs continue to meet professional standards. It validates the NP's ongoing ability to deliver high-quality care through mandatory education and clinical practice. The requirements for this process vary among credentialing bodies, depending on the specialty. Each organization establishes specific guidelines to ensure that NPs maintain their competence. Recertification programs adhere to standards set by the Accreditation Board for Specialty Nursing Certification and the National Commission for Certifying Agencies, thus ensuring their integrity and value [1].

NPs certified through the American Association of Nurse Practitioners (AANP) or the American Nurses Credentialing Center (ANCC) can recertify using two primary pathways. The first pathway is through practice hours and CE. NPs opting for this pathway must complete a minimum of 1,000 practice hours and 100 advanced practice contact hours during the five-year period. The 100 contact hours includes at least 25 pharmacology credits. Additionally, preceptorship hours can be converted into non-pharmacology CE credits. This option would allow up to 120 precepting hours to count as 25 CE credits. The other way to recertify is through successfully completing the certification exam within the five-year certification period [1].

Another example is recertification for pediatric nurse practitioners (PNPs). This is an annual process, structured over a seven-year cycle. PNPs must complete pediatric update modules and pharmacology-related activities, as outlined for the cycle [2]. Additionally, the PNCB provides guidance on credential retirement and reinstatement for practitioners who are retiring or have expired certifications [2]. Overall, staying informed with the certification body ensures compliance with the recertification process.

Besides recertification, CE is essential to stay up to date. Professional organizations provide valuable resources and programs to support these efforts. NPs can also certify in additional specialties; for example, a family nurse practitioner (FNP) can pursue certification as a psychiatric NP. There is always room for CE in the profession, and it's never too early or late to expand one's expertise. Below are some valuable resources for obtaining CE.

Continuing Education Resources for Nurse Practitioners

Resource	Website	Overview
American Association of Nurse Practitioners (AANP)	http://www.aanp.org	AANP offers a wide range of CME options: online courses, webinars, and conferences.
American Nurses Credentialing Center	http://www.nursingworld.org	ANCC offers a wide range of CME options: courses, webinars, and conferences.
Nurse Practitioner Associates for Continuing Education (NPACE)	http://www.npace.org	NPACE offers in-person and virtual conferences, as well as online courses.

(continued)

Resource	Website	Overview
UpToDate	http://www.uptodate.com	UpToDate is a clinical decision support tool that allows healthcare providers to earn CME credits as they read up on clinical content.
Board Vitals	http://www.boardvitals.com	Board Vitals provides question banks and CME activities for NPs. It is useful for preparing for board exams.
My CME	http://www.mycme.com	My CME offers a broad selection of online CME courses for various specialties and allows users to track their credits and certificates.
PESI Healthcare	http://www.pesi.com	PESI Healthcare offers a variety of CE courses, webinars, and workshops. They cover various specialties.

Resource	Website	Overview
Mayo Clinic School of Continuous Professional Development	`http://www.ce.mayo.edu`	The Mayo Clinic offers CME programs, including online and live courses. Their programs cover various topics, including primary care, specialties, and procedure-based learning.
Medscape	`http://www.medscape.com`	Medscape offers a variety of free CME opportunities in the form of articles, quizzes, videos, and webinars. They cover a broad spectrum of medical specialties.
Pri-Med	`http://www.pri-med.com`	Pri-Med offers free and low-cost CME opportunities, including online courses, live virtual events, and in-person conferences.

8.3   The Leap of Faith

By Colleen Zogby, FNP-C, PhD Candidate

At 50 years old, most people aren't considering starting over. But for me, standing at the crossroads of grief and a new chapter, it was time. I was newly widowed, my youngest were preparing for college, and I was left wondering if I had the strength to take on another risk—this time, for myself.

While my boys applied to universities, I applied too, ready to become an NP. It was daunting. When Dr. Virginia Cronin, the program director, politely asked how I thought I'd manage in a class full of students my sons' age, I responded simply, "With maturity and experience." Little did I know then that leap of faith would become one of the most fulfilling decisions of my life.

I could have stayed the course as a registered nurse. It was a safe and honorable path, but deep down, I wanted more. Nursing had already given me so much—decades of experience in the ICU, countless hours in operating rooms, and leadership skills honed from my time in the Army Nurse Reserves. There, I learned to manage not only patients but also teams and to lead with discipline, empathy, and strength. My military experience gave me an in-depth understanding of resilience, of pushing through when things got tough, and of always being prepared for the unexpected. Those leadership lessons would serve me well as I embarked on the next chapter.

So, there I was, a full-time NP student, seated next to a classmate who recognized me as his mother's friend! Still, it wasn't my age that defined me but my experience. My years in the Army, the intensive care unit, and operating room had taught me how to stand tall under pressure—a skill that carried me through the challenges of academia and beyond.

Those experiences guided me through school and now propel me forward in my practice. I am a FNP, practicing in palliative care because, for me, I know it's where I can make a meaningful difference. My journey didn't end with a diploma. A few months after graduating from Le Moyne's FNP program, I found myself seeking specialized knowledge in palliative care and stumbled upon a program at the University of Maryland, Baltimore. One email to the director, Dr. Mary Lynn McPherson, turned into a call, and soon enough, I was enrolled once again, chasing the knowledge I craved.

Today, I am a PhD candidate and still feel that pull to learn and contribute. Every day, I step into the hospital, eager to work and proud to do it. Whether I'm hosting a goals-of-care discussion, managing pain, comforting a family, or lending a hand to the bedside nurse with the simplest task, I remind them that, above all, I'm a nurse first.

I've also discovered a passion for teaching, which may be why I love my role in palliative care so much. Whether I'm educating patients and families about care options or teaching students, I find joy in sharing knowledge. I often return to Le Moyne College to lecture the FNP/DNP students on palliative care, helping to prepare the next generation of providers for the journey that lies ahead of them after graduation. Watching students grow and develop reminds me of my own path, and I'm grateful to play a part in shaping theirs.

My advice? Be a NURSE FIRST. Let your experiences mold you. Whether it's your time in the Army, the OR, the ICU, or at the bedside, those experiences will make you stronger and prepare you for any journey ahead.

Continuing Education Assignment

Goal: The goal of this assignment is to help NP students explore various CE and certification opportunities.

Assignment Instructions

Research two different CE or certification opportunities. They can be relevant to your NP specialty or exploring a new certification. Focus on identifying options that align with your career goals. Summarize the significance of these opportunities for NPs, discussing how they contribute to professional growth and clinical competency. Create a CE plan for the first year of practice, specifying at least two activities.

Rubric

Research two CE opportunities. Describe each with information on how to access (two paragraphs) 50%.

Summarize how these opportunities contribute to professional growth and clinical competency. (1–2 paragraphs) 25%

Well-defined CE plan with specific activities. 25%

8.3.1   Doctor of Nursing Practice Pathway

The DNP is a terminal degree in nursing that focuses on advanced clinical practice, leadership, and the application of evidence-based care to improve patient outcomes. Unlike a PhD in nursing, which is centered on original research, the DNP emphasizes the translation of research into practice.

Graduates of DNP programs are prepared to address complex healthcare challenges by taking on leadership roles in clinical settings [3].

A key component of a DNP program is the DNP project. Grounded in the eight DNP Essentials outlined by the American Association of Colleges of Nursing (AACN), students exhibit leadership and clinical expertise by addressing a real-world healthcare challenge [4]. This project allows students to demonstrate their ability to identify a problem, implement an intervention based on evidence-based guidelines, and evaluate the outcome. The DNP project also demonstrates how these projects can be sustained in different settings [4].

The availability of specific DNP programs often varies by state due to differences in regulatory requirements for advanced practice nursing. For instance, some states may have a higher demand for FNP programs due to the need for primary care providers, while others may emphasize specialties like psychiatric care or nurse leadership. Additionally, licensure requirements for certain specialties, such as nurse anesthetists or NPs, can vary by state, influencing the types of DNP programs offered [3].

8.3.1.1   Future of the DNP

The value of the DNP degree is also highlighted in the Future of Nursing 2020–2030 report, which points to the enhanced competencies of DNP-prepared nurses in elevating both patient care and healthcare systems [5]. The push for DNP education is further supported by emerging data, including the rapid expansion of DNP programs and their graduates, superior certification exam pass rates among DNP-prepared NPs, and the increasing diversity among DNP graduates. The AACN strongly supports the DNP as the terminal degree for advanced nursing practice and the entry point for NPs. The National Organization of Nurse Practitioner Faculties has set a goal to transition all entry-level NP education to the DNP degree by 2025 [6]. This strategic shift is well-documented and supported by compelling evidence, underscoring the DNP as the preferred degree for meeting the intricate demands of modern healthcare [6]. While it is not yet mandatory for all advanced practice nurses (APNs), this shift reflects the need for highly trained professionals who can incorporate research into clinical practice and drive improvements in healthcare delivery [3].

8.4   Entrepreneurship

As the role of DNP-prepared nurses evolves to include innovative solutions for improving healthcare systems, entrepreneurship emerges as a natural extension. It provides opportunities to pioneer new approaches and redefine the delivery of care in meaningful and impactful ways.

Entrepreneurship refers to an individual or a small group of partners who strike out on an original path to create a new business [7]. An aspiring entrepreneur actively seeks a particular business venture. Entrepreneurship in healthcare means coming up with new ideas and solutions to make healthcare better, easier to access, and more efficient. For example, one can create new medical devices, applications, or services that solve problems patients and providers face. Healthcare entrepreneurs work to bring fresh ideas to life and improve care for patients.

8.4.1 Nurse Practitioners with Entrepreneurial Skills

Entrepreneurial skills are essential for NPs to excel in various healthcare settings. These skills enable NPs to initiate their own practices, lead innovative projects, and advocate effectively for patient care and policy reforms. Entrepreneurship also offers NPs financial independence and the ability to create novel healthcare solutions. Additionally, it supports networking and collaboration, enhancing NPs' ability to establish meaningful professional relationships and expand their influence within the healthcare industry.

Beyond traditional practices, NPs can pursue entrepreneurial ventures in specialized clinical services, CE, healthcare consulting, and non-clinical fields such as writing or IT development [8]. Additionally, there are advantages of digital product businesses for NPs, highlighting the low overhead and potential for passive income. While digital products like eBooks, software, and courses offer a scalable model with minimal delivery costs, starting such a business demands planning and persistent effort [9]. It requires market research, selecting the right domain, and choosing an effective web platform.

While NPs are well-versed in clinical skills, entrepreneurship requires additional abilities such as hiring staff and managing operations. To succeed, they should employ strategies like identifying a niche, leveraging social media, and ensuring operational consistency [10]. Embracing these entrepreneurial roles enables NPs to extend their influence beyond the clinic, creating innovative solutions that can lead to improved patient outcomes and personal career satisfaction. Below are some areas of opportunity for NP Entrepreneurs.

Areas of Opportunity for NP Entrepreneurs

Idea	Description
Telehealth Services	Offering remote healthcare services through virtual consultations or telemedicine clinics.
Concierge Medicine	Providing membership-based or direct primary care services, offering personalized care with fixed fees.
Health Coaching and Consulting	Guiding individuals in wellness coaching, chronic disease management, and specialized programs like gut health initiatives.
Mobile Health Services	Operating mobile clinics or offering home visits to serve underserved or immobile patients.
Aesthetic and Wellness Clinics	Delivering aesthetic and wellness services, including Botox, weight loss programs, and other medical spa offerings.
Occupational Health Services	Partnering with businesses for corporate wellness or workplace clinics to provide onsite health services.
Educational and Training Services	Providing CE courses for healthcare professionals and educational programs for patients.
Healthcare Practice Consulting	Offering consulting services for practice management and regulatory compliance to assist other healthcare providers.

Idea	Description
Integrative and Holistic Health	Combining conventional and alternative therapies through functional medicine or holistic health services like acupuncture.
Digital Business	Digital products, including eBooks, software, and courses.

8.4.2   Barriers

NPs face several challenges when pursuing entrepreneurial roles. These include restrictive state regulations, insufficient business training in NP programs, and transition processes. Each of these factors can complicate the path for NPs aiming to leverage their expertise in innovative and autonomous ways.

8.4.2.1   Laws and Policies

One significant barrier for entrepreneurship is the variation in state laws regulating NP practice. In some states, NPs are required to have physician oversight for tasks like prescribing medications, which restricts their autonomy and independence [11]. Inadequate reimbursement policies also hinder NPs' ability to establish successful practices. NPs often receive lower reimbursement rates than physicians for providing the same services, which can threaten the financial viability of NP-led clinics. It is important to adhere to legal and ethical standards and staying within professional boundaries to maintain credibility and integrity [8]. Advocacy for reimbursement parity and collaboration with insurance companies are strategies to address this inequity [11].

8.4.2.2 Lack of Business Skills

Another major hurdle is the lack of business education in many NP programs [11]. Traditionally, programs focus on developing clinical skills and preparing students for certification and licensure. With heavy emphasis on subjects like advanced pathophysiology, pharmacology, and diagnostic reasoning, there's often little room for courses on business or practice management.

Historically, most NPs worked within established healthcare systems, where business skills were not seen as essential. As more NPs take on leadership roles or open independent practices, this gap in education is becoming more apparent. Skills like financial management, marketing, and billing are often learned on the job or through additional courses outside of formal NP education. While some programs have started to integrate elective or supplemental business courses, time constraints and competing priorities in the curriculum make widespread adoption challenging. Many NP's struggle to navigate the challenges of running their own practice without adequate knowledge of financing, strategic planning, and clinic management [11].

8.4.2.3 Commitment

For NPs aspiring to entrepreneurship, mastering strategic planning, marketing, and financial management is important. This is particularly vital in rural communities, where there are limited healthcare resources [12]. Many NPs are driven by a profound sense of duty to their communities. One NP captured the sentiment perfectly, saying, "If I'm not here, no one is. There wasn't a clinic here before." For such practitioners, running their clinics transcends mere business; it is a commitment to providing indispensable care. NPs have the unique opportunity to launch a variety of businesses that capitalize on their medical expertise and entrepreneurial drive. With appropriate tools, education, and support, NPs are well-equipped to navigate challenges, succeed as entrepreneurs, and profoundly impact their communities [12]. The following are some resources to assist NPs to pursue entrepreneurship.

Resources for Nurse Practitioners and Entrepreneurship

Organization	Website	Description
SCORE (Service Corps of Retired Executives)	http://score.org	A non-profit organization providing free mentoring and resources for small business owners. Local chapters available.
Nurse Practitioners in Business (NPB)	http://nursepractitionersinbusiness.com	Offers guidance and resources specifically for NPs interested in entrepreneurship.
American Nurses Association (ANA)	http://nursingworld.org	Provides business-related resources and support for nurses.

(continued)

Organization	Website	Description
Small Business Administration (SBA)	http://sba.gov	Offers extensive resources on starting and managing a small business. Includes help with a business plan.
Nurse Practitioner Business Owner (NPBO)	http:// npbusiness.org	Provides educational resources, workshops, and support for NPs looking to start and manage their own practices.
National Nurses in Business Association (NNBA)	http://nnba.net	Offers resources, networking opportunities, and support for nurse entrepreneurs.
The Institute for Healthcare Improvement (IHI)	http://ihi.org	Provides resources on healthcare quality improvement and practice management.

Organization	Website	Description
LinkedIn Learning	http://linkedin.com/learning	Offers courses and webinars on business management, entrepreneurship, and healthcare practice management.
Harvard Business Review (HBR)	http://hbr.org	Features articles and resources on entrepreneurship, business strategies.

8.4.3 Overview for Opening a Primary Care Practice

Opening a primary care practice as an NP is a rewarding but complex endeavor that requires research, planning, and strategic execution. The following is a general outline of actions. The initial step involves conducting market research to pinpoint the healthcare needs of the target patient population. One should assess demographics such as age, income, and prevalent health issues within that area. Also, analyzing local competition from other practices would be useful [13].

Following the research phase, the next task is to develop a comprehensive business plan. This plan should articulate the practice's mission and goals, detailing the services offered. It must include a market analysis, marketing strategy, an itemization of startup costs, and income projections. This document is vital for securing necessary funding.

Legally establishing the practice involves multiple steps. Choosing an appropriate legal entity, such as a Limited Liability Company (LLC) or corporation, as well as registering the business with the state is next. Necessary credentials, such as an Employer Identification Number from the Internal Revenue Service (IRS), NP license, National Provider Identifier, and a Drug Enforcement Administration (DEA) number for prescribing controlled substances, must be obtained [14]. Selecting and setting up a physical location that complies with ADA and health code standards is important [13].

Operational setup is the final stage before opening. This stage includes purchasing medical and office equipment and hiring staff. Developing clinical and administrative protocols for efficient practice management is also important. Marketing strategies, such as establishing a professional website, social media engagement, and community networking, will help attract patients. Continual monitoring of patient feedback supports sustained success and growth.

8.5   Entrepreneurship in Nursing

By Theresa Setter, APRN-BC, DCNP
CEO of Revitalize Dermatology & Aesthetics

Dating back to the days of Florence Nightingale, the nursing field is one of the most versatile and exciting professions one could have. In 1996, I would never have even fathomed the idea of what a nurse entrepreneur could be, nor would I have ever thought to put the two titles together. The field has evolved tremendously since the 1800s and now allows nurses autonomy as well as career options in several different specialties from school nursing to professor of nursing education or first assistant in surgery to a primary care practice owner and CEO.

Personally, I've always been somewhat of an entrepreneur; I was a paper girl for 10 years, I hustled to rake leaves and shovel the snow for the neighbors as a child for a few dollars, worked as a nanny and filed medical records for five dollars at the neighborhood doctor's office. I never would've imagined to be where I am today, and this is a brief version of the evolution of my nursing career.

I graduated in 2000 from Holy Family University and began a surgical nursing career at Thomas Jefferson University Hospital (TJUH) specializing in Cardiothoracic, transplant and trauma surgery. In 2001, I began my master's program at TJU and that culminated with a position as a first assist in open heart surgery. During my master's program, I also had two children and after a few months of being on-call decided to change my field specialty to dermatology to allow more family time.

In 2011, I relocated from Pennsylvania to New York and, after interviewing with several local dermatology practices, I decided to research the requirements for starting my own practice with a collaborating physician. Sadly, I had to forego practicing medical dermatology because I couldn't find a dermatologist willing to collaborate and so I proceeded with the aesthetic dermatology only. Having no business background, I turned to the internet on "how to write a business plan." At the time, it was a bit overwhelming because I thought I was writing a plan that had to be adhered to from start to the end of time. Might I add that my starting budget was only $20,000, which resulted in a Home Depot doorbell as my secretary, in the case that I was in an exam room when someone arrived, a personal cell phone as a telephone operator and a paper-back weekly planner as my sophisticated schedule of clients.

Three years into the growth of my med spa, I was really missing the practice of medical dermatology and signed on to work as a private contractor for a local dermatologist within my med spa location. He was not on-site while I was in the clinic and, once again, I became overwhelmed with a schedule that was not conducive to the care that I longed to provide. I continued this contracting for three years until the heavy schedule and the growth of my med spa was no longer a good business plan and I longed for change.

This is when I learned about The Nurse Practitioner Modernization Act. This Act, which greatly expanded the scope of practice for NPs, was adopted in New York State in 2015 and everything changed for me and for my practice. After several years of contracts with dermatologists, non-compete clauses, negotiations regarding compensation and being forced to see six to eight patients in an hour, the thought of change and not having to work with a collaborating physician was a very exciting one. I re-wrote my business plan to include medical dermatology within my scope of practice, took a huge risk and moved my practice to a larger location in a more visible area and hired two employees to replace my cell phone-operator and doorbell-secretary. Yes, I also invested in scheduling software and electronic medical record (EMR) to replace my daily planner.

The next hurdle was bigger than I had anticipated and involved educating insurance companies regarding the new laws and essentially begging for them to credential me for insurance participation. This took over a year, many hours on the phone, and some visits to Albany. With the help of some of our local representatives, I was granted credentialing for reimbursement from Medicare and most commercial insurance companies.

As one could imagine and as I learned, the business plan evolves with the growth and changes within the practice sometimes daily. The business plan went from being one of the most stressful parts of starting a practice to the most exciting part. I began to feel so comfortable with growth that I became a resource for other entrepreneurial NPs interested in autonomous practice, offered shadowing opportunities, and even became precepting faculty for State University of New York and Le Moyne College. Currently, I am practicing six days per month at my clinic in NY, four days per month at my clinic in Florida, and work from anywhere doing administrative duties for both practices. Both practices continue to grow despite numerous similar med spas opening. It's my belief that my practice has continued to incline due to my focus on community support and collaboration rather than a focus on competition.

If you're reading this, have a vision, and are inspired to take the entrepreneurial plunge, I would highly encourage you to do so. It may seem like an overwhelming task at the start, but the journey is very rewarding and there are endless possibilities within the field of nursing. There will be challenges, ideas that are a success and ideas that fail, as with any career, but that is all part of YOUR story. Nowadays, there are many nursing organizations that have formed that are in place to support NPs as a resource while building a practice. I'm excited to see how the field of nursing will continue to evolve and what new opportunities may arise. It is my hope to read many more of your success stories in nursing as the years progress. If you focus on your passion, you too can be your own boss.

Entrepreneurship Assignment

Objective: Construct a business plan for an NP-led venture.

Instructions: Develop a business plan for an NP-led venture. This could be a private practice, digital business, or other healthcare-related business. The plan should minimally include an executive summary, description with services, marketing, operational and financial plan. Use the above resources (Resources for Nurse Practitioners and Entrepreneurship) or other scholarly resources.

(continued)

(continued)

Rubric

Criteria	Excellent (20 points)	Good (15–20 points)	Satisfactory (10–15 points)	Needs Improvement (0–5 points)
Executive Summary	Concise and compelling summary of the plan	Adequately summarized, clear objectives	General overview with vague objectives	Incomplete or unclear summary
Business Description with Services Described	Thorough and inspiring with clear statements	Well-described, mission and vision included	Basic description and goals provided	Lacks clarity or detail, missing elements
Marketing and Sales Strategy	Innovative and fully developed strategy	Solid strategies. Some lacking information	Basic strategies outlined. Missing details	Poorly developed strategies
Operational Plan	Extensive detail on all operational aspects	Good detail, some areas not fully covered	Basic operational details covered	Many operational details missing or unclear
Financial Plan	Detailed and realistic	Minor errors or omissions	Lacks detail	Incomplete, missing data

Total: 100 points

8.6   Outcome Measures

8.6.1   Relative Value Units

Understanding the value of contributions as an NP is fundamental. This information is useful during initial contract negotiations as well as performance reviews. Relative value units (RVUs) provide a standardized way to measure the worth of healthcare services. RVUs represent the time, skill, and complexity involved in delivering specific medical services or procedures. They play a key role in determining compensation and tracking productivity across different specialties and services [15].

One way to help understand RVUs is to think of it like a scoring system that assigns value to each service an NP provides. Similar to how a car's value might be assessed like engine performance or safety components, RVUs assign value to medical services based on their complexity and the time to perform. This system ensures that services are evaluated consistently, helping to create equitable compensation for healthcare providers.

RVUs are particularly important in healthcare because they provide a fair and uniform method for calculating payments. Organizations like Medicare and private insurers use RVUs to set reimbursement rates, making it easier to balance payments across providers and specialties. This system ensures consistency. For new NPs, understanding RVUs helps to navigating compensation models, negotiating contracts, and ensuring fair pay for the services they provide.

8.6.1.1   Three Components of RVUs

RVUs are calculated based on three essential components that reflect different aspects of healthcare delivery. Work RVUs (wRVUs) measure the time, skill, and effort required to provide care. For example, a routine follow-up visit has a lower wRVU compared to managing a patient with multiple complex conditions that demands more expertise and decision-making. Practice expense RVUs account for the costs of running a practice, including office space, supplies, and employee salaries. Higher values are assigned to services that require additional resources like specialized equipment. Lastly, the malpractice RVUs factor in the cost of malpractice insurance, which varies based on the risk level of the procedure or service. Together, these three components create a standardized system to measure the value of healthcare services and ensure equitable compensation. This also allows for more efficient resource allocation.

8.6.1.2 Compensation

Many healthcare organizations use RVUs to structure compensation models, combining a base salary with additional earnings based on the RVUs a provider generates. This system not only determines bonuses and incentives but also provides a standardized way to measure and compare productivity, offering employers a clear view of the value they contribute to a practice. For new NP graduates, understanding RVUs is particularly important. It often takes up to a year to build a full patient load, so RVU targets should account for this adjustment period. By understanding how these targets align with the role and workload, realistic expectations can be set.

8.6.1.3 Conversion Factor

The conversion factor is a key component in determining compensation for healthcare services. It represents the dollar amount paid per RVU and directly impacts reimbursement for medical services or procedures. For example, if a service is assigned an RVU of 2.5 and the conversion factor is $34.89, the total reimbursement would be 2.5×$34.89, equaling $87.23.

Medicare updates its conversion factor annually based on factors like healthcare cost inflation and budget considerations, while private insurers may set their own rates. NPs should pay close attention to these rates, as they affect overall earnings and help assess whether compensation aligns with their skills and workload. Familiarity with RVUs and the conversion factor enables NPs to understand how productivity and services are valued. Whether used to calculate bonuses, measure performance, or ensure fair pay, understanding these concepts is an important step toward building a successful and fulfilling career.

NPs receive a base salary and may earn bonuses tied to the number of RVUs they generate, creating an incentive for higher productivity while ensuring that providers are compensated fairly for the complexity and time associated with their work [15, 16].

8.6.1.4   Example of RVU Calculation

The following is an example of how RVUs are used to calculate compensation for an NP working in primary care. In this scenario, the conversion factor is $40 per RVU, and the NP has a combination of office visits and minor procedures. It demonstrates how RVU-based earnings are calculated and combined with a base salary, giving a clearer picture of how productivity can translate to compensation.

Services Provided
Level 3 Office Visit: 1.50 RVUs each
Level 4 Office Visit: 2.43 RVUs each

Minor Procedure 1.00 RVU each
Monthly Productivity

Level 3 Office Visits: 60 visits × 1.50 RVUs = 90 RVUs
Level 4 Office Visits: 40 visits × 2.43 RVUs = 97.2 RVUs
Minor Procedures: 20 procedures × 1.00 RVU = 20 RVUs

Total RVUs for the Month: $90 + 97.2 + 20 = 207.2$ RVUs
Monthly Compensation

RVU Earnings: 207.2 RVUs × $40 per RVU = $8,288
Base Salary: $6,000 per month
Total Monthly Compensation: $6,000 + $8,288 = $14,288

8.6.1.5   Quantity Vs. Quality

When evaluating RVU-based compensation contracts, it's essential to strike a balance between productivity and quality care. This balance ensures patients' well-being and enhances provider satisfaction. Contracts focused solely on RVU targets tend to prioritize quantity over quality, which can lead to excessive workloads, burnout, and reduced care quality. For example, the prospect of earning an additional $20,000 annually based on RVUs might seem attractive. However, the increased demands such as longer hours spent on documentation, fewer breaks, and managing more triage calls might not be worth the financial incentives. This can often lead to provider dissatisfaction [17]. A more balanced compensation model that values quality care and promotes provider well-being would be beneficial.

Quality metrics, such as patient satisfaction scores and adherence to evidence-based care guidelines, play a critical role in maintaining a balance between productivity and care standards. According to a 2023 Medical Group Management Association poll, 47% of medical groups are now linking quality performance metrics to physician compensation. This shift reflects a growing focus on enhancing care quality alongside productivity [18]. This trend towards valuing quality is further demonstrated by the emphasis on patient-centered outcomes and adherence to evidence-based practices.

8.6.2   Clinical Performance Measures

Clinical performance measures are tools used by healthcare organizations and providers to assess the quality and effectiveness of care. These measures are customizable, allowing organizations to focus on their unique goals, such as improving chronic disease management and optimizing preventive care. For example, a primary care clinic might track the percentage of patients receiving appropriate follow-up for elevated blood pressure or adherence to diabetes management guidelines. By aligning with evidence-based practices, these measures ensure providers deliver high-quality, patient-centered care. A more standardized set of measurable criteria is Healthcare Effectiveness Data and Information Set (HEDIS) measures. These measures offer a framework for aligning provider performance with benchmarks.

8.6.2.1   HEDIS Measures

HEDIS, developed by the National Committee for Quality Assurance (NCQA), is a comprehensive set of standardized performance measures used by health plans to assess the quality of care and services provided to their members [19]. It includes over 90 measures spanning various domains of healthcare. They focus on preventive care, chronic disease management, and access to care. These measures evaluate key areas of healthcare quality, such as the effectiveness of care, access to services, and patient experience [19].

Preventive care measures, such as immunization rates and cancer screenings, are central to HEDIS. Additionally, patient experience metrics, which assess satisfaction and care quality, provide insights into patients' perceptions of their care. These insights help identify opportunities to improve communication and service delivery. Collectively, HEDIS metrics offer a robust framework for NPs to evaluate and enhance their practice.

8.6.2.2 Application

For NPs, integrating HEDIS measures into their practice provides a framework for enhancing patient care. Starting early in their careers, NPs can collect and analyze data to establish a performance baseline and identify areas for improvement. This systematic approach enables NPs to monitor their progress, refine their clinical skills, and actively participate in quality improvement initiatives. By aligning their practice with evidence-based metrics like HEDIS, NPs can demonstrate their effectiveness in various clinical settings [20]. Furthermore, patient satisfaction scores are vital as they provide insights into patients' perceptions of their care, the quality of interactions, and their overall satisfaction with the services provided [21]. These metrics are instrumental in continuous improvement and preventive strategies [22].

8.6.2.3 HEDIS Measure Example

The "Controlling High Blood Pressure" metric evaluates the percentage of adults aged 18–85 diagnosed with hypertension. Previously, the target blood pressure range was below 140/90mmHg within the measurement year. For the 2025 HEDIS update on hypertension management, changes are being introduced to align with updated medical guidelines, including a more stringent benchmark of less than 130/80mmHg [23].

In a family practice setting, an NP begins by using the EMR to identify patients diagnosed with hypertension accurately. During each patient visit, the blood pressure is measured and documented. Regular reviews of these records enable the NP to monitor the proportion of patients maintaining blood pressure levels below the threshold.

Interventions: Review and Adjust

For patients not meeting the target, the NP may implement several interventions, such as adjusting medications in accordance with guidelines. Also, the NP can provide education on lifestyle modifications, and scheduling more frequent follow-up appointments for closer monitoring. At the end of each measurement year, the NP reviews the collected data to determine the percentage of patients who have achieved the target blood pressure. This outcome serves as a benchmark for the NP's performance on the HEDIS measure. If a significant number of patients remain above the target, the NP may reassess the overall management strategy, enhance educational efforts, or tailor treatment plans more closely to individual needs.

HEDIS Measure Examples

Category	Measure	Description
Effectiveness of Care	Breast Cancer Screening	Percentage of women aged 50–74 who had a mammogram in the past two years.
	Diabetes Care: HbA1c Control	Percentage of patients with diabetes with controlled blood sugar (HbA1c < 8%).
Behavioral Health	Follow-Up After Hospitalization for Mental Illness	Percentage of discharges for mental illness with a follow-up visit within 7 and 30 days.

(continued)

Category	Measure	Description
Access/ Avail- ability wof Care	Prenatal and Postpartum Care	Timeliness and fre- quency of prenatal and postpartum visits for women giving birth.
Utilization	Hospitalization for Potentially Preventable Complications	Rate of hospitaliza- tions for conditions that could be man- aged outpatient.
Overuse/ Appropri- ateness	Appropriate Treatment for Upper Respira- tory Infection	Percentage of patients with upper respiratory infection not receiving antibiotics.

HEDIS Updates for Inclusive Care

The 2024 updates to the HEDIS focus on streamlining data collection, consolidating measures, and promoting inclusivity. For example, this includes expanding the gender-inclusive criteria for breast cancer screening and cervical cancer screening to better accommodate transgender patients. This allows health plans to assess cancer risks more accurately in this population. Additionally, the race and ethnicity stratification reporting has been broadened to include nine more measures, such as follow-up after hospitalization for mental illness and childhood immunization status, to help address health disparities. These updates reflect efforts to make HEDIS a more efficient and inclusive tool for improving healthcare quality [19].

8.6.2.4   Balancing Quantity and Quality

When measuring the productivity of NPs, it is important to consider both the quality and quantity of care they provide. Balancing these factors is key to assessing their true value in healthcare settings. Quantity can be measured through metrics like RVUs, which track the volume and complexity of services delivered. However, quality should also be evaluated based on patient outcomes, satisfaction, and adherence to clinical guidelines. Importantly, a focus solely on quantity can lead to burnout, as it places undue stress on NPs to increase their workload. This potentially compromises both their well-being and the quality of care provided. A balanced approach helps healthcare organizations achieve their goals and help prevent burnout in providers while still delivering high-quality patient care.

HEDIS Assignment

Objective:
To understand HEDIS performance measures and how to use them to improve patient care in practice.

Instructions:
Write a brief introduction summarizing HEDIS and its relevance to NP practice. Select one HEDIS measure, describe the NP would implement it in a practice setting using tools like EMRs. Outline steps to track and manage specific care components of patients. Explain how this measure would improve patient outcomes and support performance evaluations.

(continued)

(continued)
Rubric

Criteria	Excellent (90–100%)	Good (80–89%)	Needs Improvement (Below 80%)	Weight
Introduction to HEDIS	Clear and concise summary with relevance to NP practice	Good summary with minor gaps	Limited or unclear summary	30%
Application of Measure	Detailed, practical steps with clear tools and patient outcome focus	Good application with some detail missing	Lacks clear steps or focus on outcomes	50%
Clarity and Organization	Well-organized and professional tone throughout	Mostly clear with minor issues	Disorganized or lacks professional tone	20%

8.7   Interprofessional Education

8.7.1   Overview

IPE is where healthcare providers from different specialties to work in unison offering holistic, patient-centered care [24]. For new NPs, understanding the value of these collaborative partnerships is ideal. The Institute of Medicine (IOM) highlights the critical role of IPE and teamwork in enhancing patient outcomes and the quality of healthcare services [24]. Effective interprofessional collaboration fosters a synergistic approach to patient care, leveraging the unique skills and perspectives of each team member. For example, in a primary care setting, an NP may collaborate with a registered dietitian, a pharmacist, and a behavioral health counselor to manage a patient with diabetes. By integrating their expertise, the team ensures the patient receives comprehensive care, including medication adjustments, nutritional counseling, and mental health support. NPs play an important role in this collaborative model ensure holistic and well-coordinated care [25].

8.7.2   Effectiveness

IPE significantly impacts the work environment for all health professionals. A review by Medina-Córdoba et al. (2024) revealed that IPE fosters improvements in organizational climate and culture and promotes collaboration and effective communication within healthcare teams [26]. The study emphasized that the benefits of IPE align with the goals of the Quadruple Aim.

Quadruple Aim was introduced as an evolution of the widely recognized Triple Aim framework, offering a more holistic approach to improving healthcare system performance. It focuses on four key goals: reducing costs, enhancing population health, improving the patient experience, and promoting the well-being of healthcare teams. The fourth addition of well-being highlights the critical need to address burnout among providers. These priorities are essential for improving healthcare quality.

8.7.3 Safety

IPE interventions are being recognized for their potential to enhance patient safety. This is by fostering effective collaboration among healthcare professionals. Jiang et al. (2024) highlight that many patient safety incidents are rooted in poor communication and teamwork [27]. This emphasizes the value of IPE in addressing these challenges. Simulation-based learning and face-to-face methods emerged as popular approaches, showcasing IPE's versatility in engaging learners. Many interventions focused on outcomes like knowledge and attitudes rather than directly measuring patient safety incidents. These findings still suggest a meaningful connection between IPE and improved healthcare outcomes.

8.7.4 Application to Nurse Practitioners

For new NPs entering clinical practice, embracing IPE and collaboration is crucial. NPs serve as essential links within interprofessional teams, facilitating communication across disciplines and championing patient-centered care. Exposure to IPE during their training equips NPs with the skills necessary for effective teamwork and collaboration going into practice. Additionally, onboarding programs that integrate IPE principles can provide vital support, easing NPs' transition into clinical roles.

In other cases, collaboration extends to consulting with specialists and making referrals. An NP may refer a patient to a pediatric gastroenterologist for specialized procedures, ensuring access to necessary expertise. Beyond individual care, NPs also participate in community health initiatives, collaborating with public health officials, schools, and community groups to address wider health challenges. Pediatric NPs play a critical role in school health programs, working with school nurses, teachers, and administrators. This teamwork enables early identification of health issues, ensuring that children receive timely and appropriate care within the educational setting. Through these collaborations, NPs extend their impact by providing holistic care. This focus on interprofessional collaboration aligns with the objectives of the Quadruple Aim.

8.7.5 Opportunities for Future

IPE plays a pivotal role in addressing complex global challenges like climate change and advancing planetary health. By fostering collaboration across diverse disciplines and emphasizing shared values and mutual respect, IPE enables healthcare professionals to tackle issues where human and environmental well-being are deeply interconnected [28]. Interprofessional environmental health education is especially vital for achieving universal health coverage (UHC) and responding effectively to disasters. Oerther et al. (2024) emphasize that UHC relies on a strong primary healthcare system, supported by an environmentally trained workforce that includes environmental scientists, engineers, and public health nurses [28]. Together, these professionals work to mitigate environmental hazards and health crises.

Jiang et al. (2024) emphasize that IPE improves teamwork and communication but note the need for standardized ways to measure its outcomes. Developing consistent assessment methods and using creative evaluation strategies can help build stronger evidence. This would make it easier to compare IPE's effectiveness in different settings. Future research should focus on using rigorous methods, like randomized controlled trials, and include detailed outcome measures to assess IPE's long-term effects.

IPE Discussion Questions

How can NPs leverage IPE to enhance their roles in healthcare teams?

What strategies can be incorporated into NP training programs to effectively develop interprofessional collaboration skills? Provide examples of activities or approaches to help with communication and teamwork.

8.8   Snapshot of AI in Healthcare

By Charles DeSimone PhD

8.8.1   Introduction

AI has transitioned from a theoretical concept into vital technology used across various disciplines, including healthcare. Early pioneers like Alan Turing and Noam Chomsky laid the foundation for intelligent systems, shaping how AI interacts with human processes. As AI advances, particularly in healthcare, it is important to continually assess and improve both natural and artificial methods of understanding and problem-solving [29, 30]. This overview outlines AI's evolution from its early theoretical roots to its modern-day applications, emphasizing the importance of evaluating AI's role in healthcare.

8.9 Historical Foundations of AI

8.9.1 Natural Language Processing

AI's foundational ideas can be traced back to Alan Turing's "Computing Machinery and Intelligence" (1950), where he introduced the Turing test to evaluate whether machines could exhibit human-like intelligence [31]. The Turing test is a game where a person chats with an unknown partner, which could be a machine or another human. If the person can't tell if they're talking to a machine or a human, the machine passes the test. Noam Chomsky's work on language structures, such as syntax and grammar, added another layer to AI by demonstrating how human language could be processed using rule-based systems. Chomsky's theories helped develop natural language processing (NLP), a key component of AI systems that enables computers to understand and produce human language. These early contributions laid the groundwork for building intelligent systems capable of interacting with humans through language [29, 30].

8.9.2 The Turing Test and AI Verification

The Turing test remains a benchmark for assessing whether AI can mimic human behavior convincingly. As AI systems become more advanced, the lines between human-generated and machine-generated content blur, whether in text, speech, or medical diagnostics. The increasing reliance on AI in healthcare emphasizes the importance of AI outputs being accurate, timely, and indistinguishable from human expertise. For instance, AI-driven diagnostic tools now interact with patients and healthcare systems, raising the bar for both AI sophistication and medical decision-making [29].

8.9.3   Advancements in Computing Power

AI's rapid progress is not solely due to improved algorithms but also advancements in computational hardware. Technologies like tensor processing units and graphics processing units have dramatically increased the processing power available for AI tasks. These advancements are critical in healthcare, where AI systems need to process large amounts of data to provide real-time diagnostic insights. With massive clusters of these processors, capable of performing trillions of calculations per second, AI is poised to handle more complex medical tasks, such as analyzing imaging data or patient records, with increasing speed and accuracy [31].

8.9.4   Machine Learning and Transformers

Modern AI relies heavily on machine learning models, particularly transformer architectures, which have revolutionized NLP. Introduced by Vaswani et al. (2017), the transformer model enables AI systems to understand the context of language with unprecedented accuracy [32]. This innovation is essential in healthcare, where AI applications like Bidirectional Encoder Representations from Transformers (BERT) and Generative Pre-trained Transformer

4 (GPT-4) are used to analyze medical literature, support clinical decision-making, and even interact with patients. BERT excels at understanding the meaning of text by considering the context of words in both directions, making it ideal for tasks like extracting information from medical records or answering complex queries. GPT-4, a more advanced generative model, can produce coherent, human-like text and is used for tasks such as generating medical summaries, drafting patient education materials, or simulating patient interactions. These models learn from vast datasets and can perform various tasks with minimal human input, greatly enhancing healthcare workflows [32, 33].

8.10   AI Applications in Healthcare

At the 2024 European Respiratory Society (ERS) Congress in Vienna, experts discussed the growing role of AI in healthcare, focusing on both its potential benefits and the risks it poses. The US Food and Drug Administration has cleared over 600 AI-powered medical devices, reflecting AI's growing prevalence [34].

8.10.1   Patient Engagement and Operations

AI brings many advantages to healthcare. One major benefit is how it can help improve patient engagement. For example, conversational AI models can guide patients through the risks and benefits of their treatment, allowing them to take their time and ask questions. AI can also help predict the preferences of patients who can't communicate, using data like social media and medical records. This could make it easier to ensure treatments align with a patient's wishes.

Beyond improving patient engagement, AI is revolutionizing healthcare operations, such as resource management and efficiency. AI can help hospitals manage resources, such as making better decisions about bed availability, which can improve both efficiency and patient outcomes [34].

8.10.2   Predictive Modeling

AI uses different algorithms to predict medical conditions, even when data is limited. Rojek et al. (2024) introduced a hybrid model using data from 8,763 patients [35]. Logistic Regression performed well for early screenings, showing high accuracy. However, the study highlighted challenges such as small datasets and the lack of diversity in data, which can lead to bias and limit how well the results apply to different populations. To improve prediction accuracy and make AI more useful in healthcare, larger and more diverse datasets, as well as better integration into healthcare systems, are needed [35].

8.10.3   Improving Radiology and Healthcare with Advanced AI Technologies

Large Language Models (LLMs) are a type of AI that processes and generates human-like text based on the data they have been trained on. In the field of radiology, these advanced AI technologies are transforming how information is extracted from medical imaging reports [33]. Recent advancements, such as the Vicuna model, have shown to be highly effective in extracting data, offering a significant improvement over older systems. These AI models can adapt and generate more accurate analyses of radiological data. These LLMs enhance diagnostic accuracy by identifying errors and transforming free-text reports into structured formats. This not only lightens the workload for radiologists but also leads to more consistent medical records [36]. Additionally, the ability to operate these models locally on-site helps address privacy concerns, making them highly suitable for use in sensitive healthcare environments [36].

Ensuring the reliable integration of AI in healthcare remains a challenge despite its transformative potential. Models like the Large Language Model Meta AI (LLaMA), developed by D'Antonoli and Bluethgen in 2024, are addressing key concerns, including privacy and compliance in applications and research, to ensure AI technologies can be safely integrated into radiological practices [33].

For healthcare providers, integrating AI applications into clinical workflows significantly enhances diagnostic processes and improves patient care efficiency. These models handle vast amounts of data, enabling quicker and more accurate clinical decisions. However, maintaining effectiveness and accuracy requires continuous training and evaluation of AI systems in real-world clinical settings. Collaborations among healthcare providers, AI developers, and regulators are essential to align AI use with healthcare standards, promote ethical applications, and ensure the technology's long-term success [37].

8.10.4   *Robots and Computer Vision in Surgical Training*

Computer vision, a branch of AI that processes and analyzes visual data like images or videos, has exciting applications in robotic surgery. This technology, particularly through the use of convolutional neural networks (CNNs), evaluate technical skills during surgical procedures by analyzing movements and decisions made by surgeons in real time.

In a study by Yang et al. (2023), AI and computer vision were utilized to assess surgeon performance during colorectal surgeries. The focus was on the critical task of peritoneal closure, where the technology monitored precision and adherence to best practices, providing feedback that could help improve surgical outcomes [38]. The study analyzed 92 video clips of robotic surgeries and compared AI-derived metrics with human ratings using the Global Evaluative Assessment of Robotic Skills. The AI system, built on the Mask R-CNN architecture tracked and detected surgical tools during the procedures [39]. The system successfully measured key performance indicators such as tool efficiency and dexterity with both hands. The results revealed that more proficient surgeons used fewer tool movements and exhibited better bimanual coordination, closely aligning with human evaluations (Yang et al., 2023). This AI-driven approach provides objective, real-time feedback for surgical training. It offers a standardized and more precise method for assessing surgical skills. This could lead to improved training techniques for surgeons.

AI's ability to offer real-time, objective feedback could significantly reduce human error and improve the precision of skill assessments. However, there is a need for more research, with larger and more diverse datasets. This is to fully validate AI's effectiveness across different surgical procedures.

8.10.5 *Precision Medicine, Diagnostics, and Drug Discovery*

AI is making great strides in precision medicine, diagnostics, and drug discovery. Ding et al. (2023) highlighted how AI integrates multi-omics data with electronic health records

(EHRs) to create more personalized treatment plans [40]. Multi-omics data combines insights from various biological layers like genes, proteins, and metabolic processes, offering a holistic view of an individual's health. This integration allows healthcare providers to tailor treatments to an individual's genetic profile and clinical history. This improves precision and reduces the need for trial-and-error in treatment decisions. By predicting patient responses more accurately, AI not only improves clinical outcomes but also helps reduce unnecessary treatments and costs.

In medical diagnostics, AI models like deep CNNs are advancing the ability to predict critical gene functions, such as promoter and enhancer activity, which are essential for gene regulation. These AI tools enhance early disease detection and optimize diagnostic techniques like transcription-factor-based biosensors (TFBs). TFBs are specialized tools that use proteins called transcription factors to detect specific changes in gene activity, providing critical insights for early disease detection and precise diagnostics. This improves the accuracy, allowing clinicians to make quicker, more effective decisions and interventions.

AI is also revolutionizing drug discovery. Ding et al. (2023) discussed how AI models using deep learning and graph neural networks can predict enzyme activity and function, crucial for drug design [40]. These models accelerate drug development by identifying potential drug targets more quickly and optimizing metabolic pathways. AI's ability to streamline the drug discovery process not only shortens the time required to develop new treatments but also increases the likelihood of successful outcomes, creating more efficient and targeted therapies.

8.11   Key Challenges

Effectively implementing AI in healthcare requires ensuring that AI models are functional, ethical, safe, and aligned with clinical needs. This integration demands meticulous governance to manage data quality, bias, transparency, and reproducibility. These are essential to maintaining trust among healthcare providers and patients [31, 32]. Addressing data privacy concerns, particularly when managing sensitive patient information, is vital to adhere to stringent privacy regulations such as General Data Protection Regulation and Health Insurance Portability and Accountability Act [33]. These are two critical regulations that govern data privacy and security, particularly relevant in healthcare settings.

Another challenge in AI deployment is the quality of data. AI systems require access to large, high-quality datasets. However, medical data is often fragmented across various systems, leading to inconsistencies and gaps that can undermine the reliability and fairness of AI applications [31, 32].

Furthermore, successful integration of AI into clinical practice requires interdisciplinary collaboration. Clinicians, data scientists, IT professionals, and regulatory experts must work closely together. This is to ensure AI technologies not only meet clinical needs but also comply with all legal and ethical standards [32, 33]. This collaborative approach is fundamental to unlocking AI's potential in healthcare without compromising safety or trust.

8.11.1   Transparency and Explainability

A fundamental challenge in the adoption of AI within healthcare is achieving transparency and explainability. AI systems must produce outputs that are not only accurate but also comprehensible to both clinicians and patients, especially in critical decision-making scenarios. The opaque nature of many AI systems, often referred to as the "black box" problem, complicates their acceptance among healthcare professionals. When the processes behind AI-generated decisions are not transparent, it undermines the trust that clinicians and patients have in these systems. Efforts are underway to develop explainable AI that provides insights into the decision-making process, although these systems have yet to achieve full transparency, contributing to a reluctance among healthcare providers to fully trust AI recommendations [34].

8.11.2 Bias

Another significant concern is the bias inherent in many AI systems. Some AI technologies might make predictions or recommendations based on data that prioritize certain outcomes, such as survival, potentially overlooking individual patient preferences for quality of life. Moreover, since many AI models are trained on data from specific demographics, they may not perform effectively across diverse patient populations. This can result in inaccurate healthcare recommendations, which is particularly problematic in a field where diversity and personalized treatment are crucial [34].

8.11.3 Ethics and Regulatory Compliance

AI technologies must adhere to stringent ethical and regulatory standards to be effectively integrated into healthcare practices. Joshua Hatherley, PhD, underscores the importance of aligning AI use with traditional bioethical principles—autonomy, beneficence, non-maleficence, and justice. This focus on ethical considerations is essential for maintaining trust in AI applications and ensuring they contribute positively to patient outcomes [34].

8.11.4   Expanding AI Beyond Cognitive Domains

To truly revolutionize healthcare, AI must expand beyond traditional areas of intelligence, such as cognitive, affective, and psychomotor domains. AI needs to address what Romiszowski (1981) referred to as "the missing domain"— social, interactive, and interpersonal intelligence [41]. These areas are crucial for improving patient care through continuous learning, autonomous interventions, and collaboration between disciplines. Advancing AI in these domains, along with ongoing improvements in surgery and medical research, could lead to transformative impacts across healthcare and other fields.

8.12   Artificial Intelligence and the Nurse Practitioner

As a positive force in the healthcare sector, NPs are increasingly pivotal in shaping the integration of technological innovations in clinical settings. AI stands out among these advancements, offering the potential to improve effectiveness of healthcare delivery.

In a 2022 systematic review, Raymond et al. examined how NPs engage with AI-based health technologies. This review outlined the types of AI tools utilized by NPs and assessed their impact on clinical activities and performance [42]. The findings revealed that NPs employ a variety of AI applications. This includes decision support systems and predictive analytics tools. These are used across diverse settings like primary care, emergency departments, and specialties such as gastroenterology. These technologies enhance diagnostic accuracy, improve treatment outcomes, and optimize patient management. Beyond using these tools, NPs actively participate in the development and evaluation of AI systems, leveraging them to enhance decision-making, particularly in complex cases and with high-risk patients.

8.12.1   Human Insights and Challenges

Although NPs are involved in the development and use of these technologies, AI cannot replicate the unique contributions NPs bring to healthcare. NPs rely on extensive education, training, hands-on experience, and intuition to shape their clinical judgment. This foundation enables them to apply knowledge gained from working with diverse patients and cases—an ability that AI, constrained by pre-programmed algorithms, cannot achieve. Intuition, a vital element of NP practice, encompasses the ability to make decisions informed by clinical experience, pattern recognition, and an understanding of individual patient contexts. For example, an NP may recognize subtle variations in a patient's behavior or symptoms that an AI might overlook, leading to more nuanced and accurate diagnoses [43].

Additionally, NPs excel at interpersonal communication, using empathy, rapport, and touch to connect with patients. They pick up on non-verbal cues and foster an environment where patients feel comfortable sharing their concerns. This human connection often uncovers critical details about a patient's health that AI cannot access [44]. While AI can efficiently process standard cases, it struggles with complex or atypical situations requiring creative problem-solving. NPs, on the other hand, adapt to unique challenges, navigate ethical dilemmas, and incorporate patient values into care plans.

NPs are also known for their holistic approach, considering factors like lifestyle factors and stress to identify underlying contributors to symptoms. For instance, an NP might probe the impact of a patient's ibuprofen use or recent death in the family through targeted questions. These are steps the AI might not take. This ability to manage uncertainty and leverage diagnostic tools to fill information gaps highlights the adaptability and insight that set NPs apart [44, 45].

NPs require ongoing training to effectively harness these technologies. Future research should prioritize empirical studies to better understand AI adoption and its long-term implications for clinical practice. By addressing these areas, AI can be seamlessly integrated into healthcare, maximizing its benefits for all.

8.13   Conclusion

AI is transforming healthcare, providing significant opportunities, and introducing complex challenges. NPs are at the forefront of integrating AI into clinical practice, utilizing tools like predictive analytics and decision support systems. This is to enhance diagnostic precision and optimize workflows. AI adoption should be accompanied by continuous education, ethical oversight, and interdisciplinary collaboration. This is to address concerns such as data privacy and the risk of technological dependency.

As healthcare progresses towards a technology-driven future, NPs are essential in balancing the benefits of AI with the necessity of compassionate, human-centered care. Their unique blend of clinical expertise, intuition, empathy, and holistic approach is indispensable. NPs are key to harnessing AI's full potential while ensuring that patient care remains human and individualized [46, 47].

Case Scenario for Group Discussion

A 50-year-old woman with a history of hypertension and hypothyroidism presents with recurrent headaches, fatigue, and digestive issues. She notes that these symptoms do not follow a clear pattern but are accompanied by increased work-related stress and sleep difficulties.

Discussion Analysis of AI Diagnostic Tools
When utilizing an AI diagnostic algorithm, it might identify common conditions associated with her symptoms, such as migraines, tension-type headaches, or irritable bowel syndrome. This identification is based on statistical patterns and clinical guidelines. However, AI systems can struggle with the subtleties and complexities of human conditions. In this scenario, the algorithm might overlook the possible impact of the patient's work stress and specific environmental

(continued)

(continued)

factors that exacerbate her symptoms. AI's reliance on structured data may also lead to misinterpretations of her subjective symptom descriptions, such as "recurrent headaches" or "digestive issues." This can result in missing critical nuances that a human clinician would likely investigate.

Discussion Questions

What are the advantages of using AI diagnostic tools in identifying common medical conditions based on symptoms like headaches and fatigue?

What limitations does AI face in integrating subjective patient data and environmental factors into its diagnostic process?

How could these limitations affect the accuracy of diagnoses in complex cases, and what role do NPs play in bridging these gaps?

8.14   Fostering the Future

By Deborah Clarey FNP-C, RNFA

Precepting is incredibly rewarding; it's my way of giving back and nurturing the next generation of NPs. When you precept an NP student, you foster growth not only in the student but also in yourself as a preceptor. It encourages the development of new strategies and concepts, and, combined with years of experience, enhances patient care and decision-making. Watching a new NP graduate and succeed builds lasting collaborations and friendships. This creates a bond that strengthens over time. It's crucial to support and motivate these new NPs, as it fosters a lifelong commitment to compassionate patient care.

I have been an NP for 25 years. My career began in Gastroenterology and Hepatology, and after many fulfilling years, I pursued further education to become a first assistant in the operating room, working in a cardiothoracic surgery specialty. Now, I'm thriving in family practice, where I've shifted my focus to holistic, patient-centered care. This transition has allowed me to engage with patients on a deeper level, promoting not just their physical health but their overall well-being. This journey has only deepened my appreciation for precepting and the lasting impact it has on the profession.

8.15   Growth of Nurse Practitioners

The NP profession continues to experience significant growth, driven by the rising demand for high-quality, patient-centered care [48]. NPs are currently the fastest-growing profession in the United States, with the US Bureau of Labor Statistics projecting a 46% increase in employment between 2021 and 2031 [46, 48]. Several factors contribute to this surge, including an aging population and shortage of primary care physicians. Furthermore, many US states have expanded NPs' practice authority, enabling them to provide a broader range of healthcare services independently. NPs also have the flexibility to specialize in various fields, such as family practice, pediatrics, women's health, mental health, and more. These diverse specializations further solidify the NPs essential role in healthcare delivery [48, 49].

The AANP has taken a leading role in advancing the NP profession internationally and worldwide to enhance patient care and address global healthcare challenges [50]. This is being done through programs such as the International Committee, the International Advanced Practice Nurse Ambassador Program, and the AANP International Specialty Interest Group. The AANP has provided NPs with access to essential education, training, and resources. These initiatives aim to support the global NP community by cultivating collaboration.

8.15.1   International Membership

To further its outreach, AANP introduced international membership options in 2021. This initiative reduces financial barriers by offering more accessible membership to NPs in economically diverse regions [50]. International members gain access to AANP's comprehensive resources, including the CE center and various clinical tools for advancing skills and competencies. This initiative also fosters global collaboration by connecting NPs worldwide. It creates a platform for sharing knowledge and supporting the mission of delivering high-quality, patient-centered care.

8.15.2   Global Networking and Contributions to Healthcare

By welcoming international members, AANP is strengthening the global NP community and highlighting the critical role NPs play in addressing healthcare disparities, particularly in underserved regions. With over 385,000 NPs in the United States, this expansion aligns with global trends to integrate APNs into healthcare systems worldwide [50].

These efforts reflect a broader commitment to improving access to care and addressing health inequities on a global scale.

NPs are making significant contributions to healthcare systems worldwide, addressing unique challenges and enhancing access to quality care. In New Zealand, Māori NPs lead culturally guided initiatives to improve health outcomes for Māori communities. Collaborative events, such as the Marae Noho (a two-day meeting), have facilitated research and policy discussions tailored to their cultural needs [51].

In China, the roles of NPs and APNs have evolved to address critical challenges, such as provider shortages and the growing prevalence of chronic diseases. Supported by organizations like the International Council of Nurses and the Global Academy of Research and Enterprise, China has implemented key initiatives to advance nurse education and leadership. This aligns with the World Health Organization's goals for primary care improvement. Notable programs include the "Specialist Qualification Certification Nurse" project, introduced in 2003, and a standardized training program launched in 2005. These initiatives have formalized APN roles in specialized areas like intensive care, emergency services, and diabetes management. This is enabling nurses to manage complex cases and expand healthcare accessibility across the country [52].

In September 2024, NPs from around the globe convened at the 13th International Council of Nurses/Nurse Practitioner/Advanced Practice Nurse Network Symposium, held in the Scottish Highlands in Aberdeen, UK [51]. Themed "Advanced practice nursing: an invaluable investment for global health," this symposium functioned as an exciting nucleus for collaboration, discussion, and exploration of future trends in nursing practice. This assembly exemplified the significant opportunities that bolster the influence of NPs on global health initiatives and aid in crafting a healthier, more equitable world.

8.16   Conclusion

In conclusion, the trajectory of NPs is a testament to their growing influence in shaping the future of healthcare. NPs are not only expanding their roles within traditional settings but also embracing entrepreneurial opportunities that promote innovative solutions. Positioned at the intersection of clinical expertise and technological advancements, such as artificial intelligence, NPs are driving transformative changes. Their commitment to IPE fosters collaboration among diverse healthcare professionals. As the profession moves toward requiring a doctorate degree for entry into practice, NPs will continue to lead with significant growth and profound impact.

References

1. American Association of Nurse Practitioners (AANP) (2024). Professional development & recertification guidelines.
2. Pediatric Nursing Certification Board (PNCB) (2024). CPNP-PC recertification. https://www.pncb.org/cpnp-pc-recertification#:~:text=Recert%20is%20annual%2C%20but%20over,Tracker%20before%20starting%20your%20application.requirements (accessed 22 October 2024).
3. American Association of Colleges of Nursing (2022). DNP education. https://www.aacnnursing.org/students/nursing-education-pathways/dnp-education (accessed 21 October 2024).

4. American Association of Colleges of Nursing (2019). The doctor of nursing practice: current issues and clarifying recommendations. https://www.aacnnursing.org/Portals/0/PDFs/Position-Statements/DNP.pdf (accessed 1 November 2024).

5. National Academy of Medicine (2021). *The Future of Nursing 2020–2030: Charting a Path to Achieve health Equity.* Washington, DC: The National Academies Press https://doi.org/10.17226/25982.

6. National Organization of Nurse Practitioner Faculties (2023). Reaffirming the DNP as the terminal degree for nurse practitioners. https://cdn.ymaws.com/http://www.nonpf.org/resource/resmgr/dnp/04_12_23_reaffirming_the_dnp.pdf (accessed 1 November 2024).

7. Stanford Online (2004). What is entrepreneurship?. https://online.stanford.edu/what-is-entrepreneurship (accessed 1 December 2024).

8. Phillips, B.C. (2020). What kind of business can a nurse practitioner start? Business question of the week. YouTube. https://www.youtube.com/watch?v=-acrHDMKoV8 (accessed 1 November 2024).

9. Hofmann, J. (2020). How to start a digital product business. NPBusiness. https://npbusiness.org/how-to-start-a-digital-product-business/#more-7617 (accessed 21 December 2024).

10. Scala, E. (2020). Nurse practitioners turned entrepreneurs: How NPs are changing the world. Health eCareers. HealtheCareers.com (accessed 21 November 2024).

11. Sharp, D.B. and Monsivais, D. (2014). Decreasing barriers for nurse practitioner social entrepreneurship. *J. Am. Assoc. Nurse Pract.* 26 (10): 562–566. https://doi.org/10.1002/2327-6924.12126.

12. Guo, K.L. (2009). Core competencies of the entrepreneurial leader in health care organizations. *Health Care Manag (Frederick).* 28 (1): 19–29. https://doi.org/10.1097/HCM.0b013e318196de5c. PMID: 19225332.

13. U.S. Small Business Administration (2024). Market research and competitive analysis. U.S. Small Business Administration. https://www.sba.gov/business-guide/plan-your-business/market-research-competitive-analysis (accessed 21 November 2024).

14. Bagley, C.E. (2018). *The Entrepreneur's Guide to Law and Strategy*, 5e. Boston: Cengage Learning.
15. Buppert, C. (2021). *Nurse Practitioner's Business Practice and Legal Guide*, 7e. Burlington: Jones & Bartlett Learning.
16. Medical Group Management Association (2023). MGMA Data-Dive cost and revenue survey. https://www.mgma.com/data/landing-pages/mgma-datadive-cost-revenue-survey (accessed 20, December 2024).
17. GoodRx (2024). Relative value units (RVUs) and burnout. GoodRx. https://www.goodrx.com/hcp-articles/providers/relative-value-units-rvus-burnout (accessed 21 December 2024).
18. MDLinx (2023). Physician compensation 2023: the good, the bad, and the ugly. https://www.mdlinx.com/exclusive/physician-compensation-2023-the-good-the-bad-and-the-ugly (accessed 21 December 2024).
19. National Committee for Quality Assurance (2023). HEDIS 2024 volume 1: technical specifications. NCQA Publications (accessed 2 December 2024).
20. Leatherman, S. and Berwick, D.M. (2020). Accelerating global improvements in health care quality. *JAMA* 324 (24): 2479–2480. https://doi.org/10.1001/jama.2020.17628.
21. HCAHPS (2023). Hospital consumer assessment of healthcare providers and systems. www.hcahpsonline.org (accessed 2 December 2024).
22. Melnyk, B.M. and Fineout-Overholt, E. (2019). *Evidence-Based Practice in Nursing & Healthcare: A Guide to Best Practice*, 4e. Philadelphia: Wolters Kluwer.
23. NCQA (2023). Proposed new measure for HEDIS® MY 2025. https://www.ncqa.org/wp-content/uploads/02.-BPC-E.pdf (accessed 22 October 2024).
24. Institute of Medicine (2015). *Measuring the Impact of Interprofessional Education on Collaborative Practice and Patient Outcomes*. Washington, DC: The National Academies Press.
25. Hamric, A.B., Hanson, C.M., Tracy, M.F., and O'Grady, E.T. (2014). *Advanced Practice Nursing: An Integrative Approach*, 5e. St. Louis: Elsevier.
26. Medina-Córdoba, M., Cadavid, S., Espinosa-Aranzales, A.F. et al. (2024). The effect of interprofessional education on the work environment of health professionals: a scoping review. *Adv. Health Sci.*

Educ. 29 (5): 1463–1480. https://doi.org/10.1007/s10459-023-10300-4.

27. Jiang, Y., Cai, Y., Zhang, X., and Wang, C. (2024). Interprofessional education interventions for healthcare professionals to improve patient safety: a scoping review. *Med Educ Online.* 29 (1): 2391631. https://doi.org/10.1080/10872981.2024.2391631.

28. Oerther, D.B., Oerther, S., and Dyjack, D.T. (2024). The urgent need for interprofessional environmental health education to achieve universal health coverage, even in disasters. *Environ Sci Technol Lett.* 11 (11): 1144–1146. https://doi.org/10.1021/acs.estlett.4c00756.

29. Turing, A. (1950). Computing machinery and intelligence. *Mind* 59 (236): 433–460.

30. Chomsky, N. (1957). *Syntactic Structures.* The Hague: Mouton.

31. Next Platform (2024). So who is building that 100,000 GPU cluster for XAI?. https://www.nextplatform.com/2024/07/30/so-who-is-building-that-100000-gpu-cluster-for-xai/ (accessed 19 August 2024).

32. Vaswani, A., Shazeer, N., Parmar, N. et al. (2017). Attention is all you need. *Adv. Neural Inf. Proces. Syst.* 30. https://doi.org/10.48550/arXiv.1706.03762.

33. D'Antonoli, T.A. and Bluethgen, C. (2024). A new era of text mining in radiology with privacy-preserving LLMs. *Radiol Artif Intell.* 6 (4): e240261. https://doi.org/10.1148/ryai.240261.

34. Callari, M. (2024). Experts weigh benefits and risks of AI in medicine at ERS congress. *Medscape Medical News.*

35. Rojek, I., Kotlarz, P., Kozielski, M. et al. (2024). Development of AI-based prediction of heart attack risk as an element of preventive medicine. *Electronics* 13 (272): https://doi.org/10.3390/electronics13020272.

36. Summers, R.M. et al. (2023). Feasibility of using the privacy-preserving large language model vicuna for labeling radiology reports. *Radiology* .

37. Gertz, R.J. et al. (2024). GPT-4 in radiology: enhancing accuracy in error detection. *Radiology* 309 (1): e231147.

38. Yang, J.H., Goodman, E.D., Dawes, A.J. et al. (2023). Using AI and computer vision to analyze technical proficiency in robotic

surgery. *Surg. Endosc.* 37 (8): 3010–3017. https://doi.org/10.1007/s00464-022-09781-y.

39. He, K., Gkioxari, G., Dollár, P., and Girshick, R. (2017). Mask R-CNN. *Proc IEEE Int Conf Comput Vis.* 2961–2969. https://doi.org/10.1109/ICCV.2017.322.

40. Ding, N., Yuan, Z., Ma, Z. et al. (2024). AI-assisted rational design and activity prediction of biological elements for optimizing transcription-factor-based biosensors. *Molecules* 29 (3512): https://doi.org/10.3390/molecules29153512.

41. Romiszowski, A.J. (1981). *Designing Instructional Systems: Decision Making in Course Planning and Curriculum Design.* London: Kogan Page.

42. Raymond, L., Castonguay, A., Doyon, O., and Paré, G. (2022). Nurse practitioners' involvement and experience with AI-based health technologies: a systematic review. *Appl. Nurs. Res.* 66: 151604. https://doi.org/10.1016/j.apnr.2022.151604. PMID: 35840270.

43. Benner, P. (1984). *From Novice to Expert: Excellence and Power in Clinical Nursing Practice.* Boston: Addison-Wesley Publishing Company.

44. Bodenheimer, T. and Sinsky, C. (2014). From triple to quadruple aim: care of the patient requires care of the provider. *Ann. Fam. Med.* 12 (6): 573–576.

45. Shanafelt, T.D. and Noseworthy, J.H. (2017). Executive leadership and physician well-being: nine organizational strategies to promote engagement and reduce burnout. *Mayo Clin. Proc.* 92 (1): 129–146.

46. Obermeyer, Z. and Emanuel, E.J. (2016). Predicting the future—big data, machine learning, and clinical medicine. *N. Engl. J. Med.* 375 (13): 1216–1219.

47. Topol, E.J. (2019). High-performance medicine: the convergence of human and artificial intelligence. *Nat. Med.* 25 (1): 44–56.

48. U.S. Bureau of Labor Statistics (2023). Occupational outlook handbook: nurse practitioners. https://www.bls.gov/ooh/healthcare/nurse-anesthetists-nurse-midwives-and-nurse-practitioners.htm (accessed 22 October 2024).

49. American Association of Nurse Practitioners (2023). Nurse practitioner profession grows to 385,000 strong. https://www.aanp.org/news-feed/nurse-practitioner-profession-grows-to-385-000-strong (accessed 21 December 2024).

50. DeSimone, M.E. and Messner, L. (2024). The international Nurse practitioner. *J. Am. Assoc. Nurse Pract.* 36 (11): 597–598.

51. NP Conferences Scotland (2024). Collaborative efforts in advanced nursing practice. https://www.icn.ch/events/npapn-network-conference-2024 (21 November 2024).

52. Zhang, Y. (2024). Development status of advanced practice nurses in China and abroad: A review. *Int J Public Health Med Res.* 2 (1): 1–14. https://doi.org/10.62051/ijphmr.v2n1.06.

Index

Nurse Practitioner: Transition Guide, First Edition. Sara L. Gleasman-DeSimone.
© 2025 John Wiley & Sons, Inc. Published 2025 by John Wiley & Sons, Inc.

Printed and bound by CPI Group (UK) Ltd, Croydon, CR0 4YY

28/10/2025

14762266-0001